BEING DISABLED IS NOT INABILITY

AMUSA ABDULATEEF

AUTHOR OF 'WORDS ARE ABSOLUTELY POWERFUL'

DEDICATION

This book is dedicated to all who are physically handicapped but are role models in wealth and employment generation across the world.

ACKNOWLEDGEMENT

All appreciation is to the Almighty Creator that bestows on me the knowledge to write for the growth of humanity and the nations. The sources of inspirations to write on different problems-solving national and global issues are amazing and no doubt a gifted from the Almighty.

I started my profound gratitude to Oloye**Yemi Ogunyemi,**retired veteran journalist of 'Tanbalaya' fame of Nigerian Television Authority, Ibadanwhose invitation to me to be at an award ceremony for the disable at a function pushed me into writing about disable and their potentials to be wealth creators instead of being human liabilities on the roads and streets. As usual and eternally, I shall never fail to salute the courage and supports of immense value from my spouse in the person of **Joy Kudirah Adunni nee Oladipupo** and ourlively children, **Abdulazeez Ayomide** and **Sheriffdeen Ayokunmi.** They are all greats in values.

May Almighty God eternally bless the souls of my beloved and irreplaceable ever caring and loving parents (of blessed memory).The level of education that I attained which is being used to proffer solutions to issues is sourced from their financial, inspirational and spiritual supports. Again and again, may their souls be pleased with till eternity.

Surveyor **Abdulrahmon Abubakar** of Geopics consult, Nigeria is always outstanding and distinct in his contributions in all my publications. I cannot forget to identify with **Alhaji Bayo Azeez** of the department of health, Ministry of Health, Oyo State for his philanthropic and moral supports of inestimable values.

I shall eternally reference to the parental supports of the likes **Mrs. Anike Abe** and her hubby, **Pastor Abe, Mr. Olabayo Olafusi, Mrs. Tomilayo Laniya** of Bloom Heights Foundation group of schools, **Mrs. Felicia Modupe Adeleke** of Nickdel group of schools,**Alhaji** and **Alhaja Rafat Idowu-Kunle Sanni** among others. Accept my eternal appreciations.

A lot of inspiration was got from the streets where the disable risk their lives while scampering for free gifted from the charity-givers. Close look shows that many of them have lost hope of self-sustenance. And this paves the way for the thinking for them in line of the wealthy disable in other saner climes. I can say that the outward disposition is inevitable guide towards compiling this for the sake of humanity and the group of beings living with one disability or the others.

<u>PREFACE</u>

Nations have very high number of people living with disabilities in one form or the other. The number of those born with disabilities is too insignificant small to the very large from the self-inflict as a result of avoidable accidents, epidemics from dirty environments and depression. In this clime, being physically challenged has become a license to beg for alms in the broad daylight without shame. A large percentage of people living with liabilities that are stark illiterates and hopeless of their situations has been truly abandoned by their families who are also living hand to mouth as a result of the abject poverty in the poorly run economy. Those who have victims of failed promises from the families, friends and governments have become destitute and public nuisance. It is sad to have many who are nursing mothers and girl-mothers procreating for unknown fathers. Many bargain for children from the poor, ignorant, docileand grossly irresponsible parents on monetary negotiations to use the innocent children most especially babies as a bait to whip up sentiment and gain empathy from the target charity or alms givers. In the clusters of beggars very near to places of worship are innocent babies wrap at the backs of the beggar mothers. All dress in tartar clothes to enjoy sympathy. The social miscreants and the future human liabilities being bred on the streets have become addition to the out of school children. It is a public nuisance watching many beggars with certain disabilities singing captivating songs to beg for alms. If sonorous songs can be sung to attract passersby who can dole out a little as alms, what could be the financial reward if the beggar with captivating voice and song is formally produced at a music studio. A closer look at the beggars on our streets shows that most of them have raw talents waiting for exploiters and promoters.

Every physically strong man can become handicapped at any time especially as a result of accidents on the roads happening on our bad roads every day. If the accident victims have their hands and legs amputated, the defect on the body has turned such into deformed. Unfortunately, in the poor climes, the beggars are treated with scorn. Some even cast spells on money before such is given to the beggars. This is insulting to the people. Had the leaders planned over their welfare, would this kind of nonsense be happening to them?

Contrary to the poor inhuman treatment on the beggars who are major physically challenged in the nation, there are lessons to learn from the other nations that respect human rights. At the sane climes, especially the advanced economies, there is no difference between the disable and the able body persons in the societies. In fact, there is plan ahead of time and situation. This is the reasons for the ambulance at every street waiting for the accident victims that need urgent medical attention. At those environments, all persons have their rights protected. Nobody should infringe on other people's right regardless of the challenges such has. In the said clime, the think tanks think outside the box on how to make provision of all the citizens in the nation. 'A sauce for goose is a sauce for gander' according to the popular maxim is the right proverb to use. The constitution protects the sanctity of the citizens particularly those who have physical and mental challenges. In the poor nation where leaders hardly make enough provision for the citizens with no deformity, the people living with disabilities have lost in the national plan. As a result of the failure of leadership to play equality, justice and fairness as enshrined in the national constitution, a large chunk of these people are left at the mercy of chance. They roam the streets begging for sustenance from the well-wishers. By this, they have resigned to fate and pick up begging as a trade. This trend of being human liabilities must change. The people with deformities could be transformed into human assets like their counterparts.

<u>**LET THE AUTHOR SPEAK**</u>

The economic realities of today show that businesses are being run on debt leverage. Many business owners are running on the basis of deficit financing where the expenditures are intentionally jerked up (greater) than the revenue in order to boost the economy from the level of decline and lower the unemployment hence increasing jobs and circulate wealth. The managers of the economy, like investors, reflate the declining economy suffering from low internally generated revenues by disposing assets and could also adopt the former (deficit financing). In some cases especially during the inflation period, government shall deflate the economy through measures such as decreasing of the costs of production and wages and the investors have cheap logistic and lower costs of production. In a declining economy, if the debt leverage where deficit financing (<u>expenditures are greater than the revenue, Internally generated revenues and the foreign earnings</u>)to boost the declining economyhas been used for years to sustain the budget and deficit spending is applicablewhere government has to engage in massive **borrowing,**locally or internationally, to fund all the critical sectors in life and business-impacting projects. This shouldbe the order of the day as a result of the deficit and decayed social infrastructure. Failure to do so, the gross domestic products shall decline to meet the demands of the citizens, abled and disabled especially those that are active not to talk of the passive population-the persons living with disabilities (PLWDs).

In retrospect, the deficit in income, (as a result of low sales, low earning, as a result of the internal and external factors) to the coffers of the nation has made it hard for the government to have adequate plan on the virile populace not to talk of the increasing number of dependents from the jobless and hopeless people among those persons living with disabilities in the nation. Failure of the nation to have running and viable economy has thrown families into depression which is a primary cause of disability. According to the National Bureau of Statistics (NBS) published 2016 research reports on depression in 2018, one out of five Nigerians is living with depression and 28% has chronic depression. By the inability to cure depression with countless other causes, the number of the citizens that would become disabled from the use of antidepressants and injections, those whose behaviours could turn them losing parts of the body to become disable increases by the day. The drunken drivers, the angry husbands that pounce on their wives battery them for insignificant issues, the impoverished and frustrated parents who maltreat or abandon the children for inability to offset their bills and the likes are path towards pushing the vulnerable to commit suicide or maim themselves. All the societal disorders emanating from rudderless leadership at the position of authorities at home, office and the nation are roadmap to disabilities. With these in view, the stakeholders should brace up to tackle the menace of anticipated increasing numbers of persons that could be living with disabilities by planning ahead for them.

By the studies of the people in Nigeria environment on regional basis, there are wealthy and influential persons among those with one form of deformity or the others and also the millions who are having one disability or the other including those who feign being disabled that have turned themselves into human liabilities. Cultural, religion and business environments have added to the proliferation of beggars from the persons living with one disability or the other in the streets. Deform babies are thrown out to the dump by heartless mothers making the disability gets worse if such is able to survive by stroke of chance later in life. A disability that must have been corrected at the early stage by surgery by indigent parents who did not bother to seek assistance from the social welfare ministry, the philanthropists, faith-based institutions, social clubs and the charity-based organizations could grow to become an impossible mission to correct again. Lack of family planning or the making of babies outside marriage especially from illegal affairs has also produced persons living with disabilities in the society. It is onus on the government and other stakeholders in the growing of the numerical strength of the nation to sensitize and support the citizens including the charity organizations to wake up on the primary responsibility and hence work on how to make gains from the begging populace through series of motivations and tasks in order to change their orientation from being liabilities into human assets. In the business environment that is not conducive for businesses to thrive, financial losses are recorded and the balance sheet of companies would always be red. By this downturn from the zero returns on capital employed to run businesses as a result of low patronage and high costs of production, jobs loss become the order of the day. By jobs loss, the number of the dependents soars, the disposable income goes south and the standard of living becomes poorer. The hardship on the people would push many who have been on the 'payroll' of the previously working population (recently sacked) into the streets to beg for sustenance. Among the population are those that required special attention before the economic downturn who are those having one defect or the other as challenges. For every right thinking person, for any economy to be boosted, all the citizens must add inputs to have growing national outputs in gross domestic products. By the word 'all', we mean <u>all without exemption</u> regardless of the physical body defects, age, race, marital status, social status, faith, academic qualification, social affiliation, political ideology or level of intelligence and exposure. We have inputs and roles to play towards boosting the economy and raise the standard of living of ourselves. With this in mind, we have done much on the people without any form of disabilities on different published books on entrepreneurial development; it is high time our lens focused on the other side towards adding right values to the socio-economic sectors and rid our streets of beggars who are potential human assets. The persons living with disabilities must have their personalities redeemed in order to discover their invaluable resources.

In retrospect, by what life has taught man in history, the creature is in transition. Life is in phases and in a transition. There is no permanent status but changes and evolutions. Statistics show that a very large percentage of people living with disabilities are not disabled by births. The inability of the midwives and the doctors could lead to disabilities; dearth of right delivery facilities at the hospitals could pave the way to disabilities; poor handling of delivery of babies is also a way to have babies with disabilities. Brief and protracted illness including the old-age related diseases could paralyze the limbs or defect the senses. For babies, the six child-killer diseases always paralyse and cripple the child if such escape infant death. Contaminated water, soil and air could lead to epidemics from the water borne, air borne diseases resulting into disabilities if not properly managed by the health service departments and workers. Many a man that is born with able body (healthy, strong limbs and sound faculties) should anticipate becoming deformities or defects by unanticipated situations in life such as accidents, self-inflict or external attacks like epidemics, wars and spiritual attacks. The latter takes the largest percentage of the people with living disabilities. Though, there are natural or inborn disabilities, everyone has a challenge or the other. If the challenges man faces is used to define disability, then every man is a disable or could be categorized as either physically or mentally challenged. By the biting of the micro and macro economy, many who intentionally abort unwanted pregnancies through the use of drugs end up birthing disable or deform babies. The harsh economy has pushed the heartless mothers to throw the innocent babies to the bush or drainage to be feasted upon by insects, pest and animals. By chance, if such survives, he or she could be infected by strange diseases that could turn him or her diseased. In many cases, the deform babies are intentionally abandoned by the mothers at hospitals or at the dump for prey to feast upon. Inability to pay the medical bills could result in keeping a diseased baby at home which will later result in the defects of the body or the malfunctioning of the senses. Ignorance could lead many inexperienced young mothers to administer non-prescribed drugs or patronize quack nurses for medical attention for their sick babies which could result in the disable of any part of the body. At my teens, I suffered to hell with malaria which almost deformed the functions of my brains in form retardation and slow learning at a period before I picked up again. The illicit use of hard drugs has turned many into a disable overnight. Many questions used to come to my mind. If a physically strong person becomes a physically handicapped as a result of avoidable accidents or preventable epidemics of diseases, would he resign his fate to become beggar on the street? Should he throw aside his reputation, integrity and good name to beg for alms in order to sustain his needs?

Nay, the journey to the disability should be a turning point to start afresh. A road starts where a road ends. There should be new will to have new way. As a pious person, everything in life is for a purpose. The dusk sneaks in when the dawn is here. People who feign disabilities start building false personalities when they are financially and economically dependents. Some join the bandwagon of street beggars after understudied the 'professional beggars' who have become wealthy from the alms received from the charity-givers. In a sane society, beggars are nuisance to the public. A sane government that cherishes manpower and quality citizens to increase outputs would think outside the box to transform the people living with disabilities into human assets from the level of human liabilities. It is not the sole responsibility of the government but all the stakeholders including the 'beggars' themselves. A disable should think outside the box to avoid being enlisted among the human liabilities and burdens to the families, friends, residents and the government. In a nation that is dreaming of prosperity, all the citizens should be proud contributors positively. Human liabilities are those who never add values to the nation but are parasites to the people and their hard earned wealth. The beggars are not adding to the Gross Domestic Products (GDP) but rather deplete the outputs from demand for free gifts. By this, the shared outputs are inadequate for the people making the life more costly and harsh for all. In the poor nations where the loss of employment is rising by the day, many who feign disability flood the streets to 'steal' from the innocents. We use the word 'steal' instead of 'fraud' because the art of begging under the guise of being a physically handicapped is a 'stealing by trick' in the crime record parlance. The nation that permits begging on the streets is discouraging hard work and increasing national output. And if the Gross Domestic Products (GDP) are low, how much of the income shall be earmarked for the sectors in the economy? The World Bank (WB) and the other development agencies suggested that a large portion of the GDP should be budgeted for education, health and social infrastructures to develop the nation especially the manpower. A friend once travelled to Tripoli in Libya during the regime of Moamer Ghadafi. He was surprised when a cripple man on the wheel chair rejected the offering offered him as a charity. It has been a custom of the people from Nigeria to dole out charity especially to those living with the physical disability meet on the roadsides. One can see the two geographic and cultural environments of the people living with disabilities. In the former, they are treated as complete persons unlike the other that ridicule the physically challenged by paying alms to them instead of providing them with the right to safety fund on monthly basis. It is our belief that they are begging for alms. The utterance from the cripple man was that he was on his way to the government house to collect his monthly salary like others who were disabled. He used an Arabic word 'haram' meaning illegal or forbidden for the 'charity' from the friend.

Ironically, if people with disabilities are registered in a payroll for social fund as safety net every month, corruption would not allow the actual beneficiaries to have the meager amount on the actual date. Secondly, the payers may have slashed the actual amount budgeted by the government. Thirdly, many who are not living with any disability may feign being one. Fourthly, we can find situation where a disabled collect in multiples. Studies and interviews confirmed that there are beggars among the people who genuinely living with disabilities that have become 'bureau de change operator' and 'bank' who provide low denominations to the customers for a percentage. Along the roads are 'bankers' among the persons living with disabilities to the corrupt security agents on the road whose personal desire beside the busy road is how to collect bribes from the motorists. The begging disabled person at the pedestrian is the bank of the corrupt security agents. The worst case is the conversion of people with deformity into gang and conspirators who connive to perpetrate criminal activities. They are active partners of the armed gangs terrorizing the nation. Trusting someone living with disabilities is a risk at the moment. In my community some years ago, there was a farmer who was cripple and in control of large scale cocoa farms. He had three wives and many children in his one story 16-room building as at the time I was living at the settlement. From the income from his cocoa farms, he was able to educate his children to tertiary institutions and financial responsible to his wives from the flamboyant lives of the wives under a roof. Since the time, I knew that no man is a liability. Every man is endowed and only required to discover his talent and horn his skill for patronage instead of throwing to the dustbin his integrity, honour, respect, reputation and dignity by begging to survive. To produce economic and financial independent persons regardless of the ability and disabilities, all stakeholders must involve themselves. We have roles to play till eternity starting from the government. For instance, if a responsible government is able to have basic plan on the provision of the basic needs (housing, feeding, clothing, security, easy communication, effective transportation and quality health services) for the people living with one disability or the other, then the nation has created the right environment for the people to be productive. Every preparation to save the beggars who are illiterates and those who are literates is towards transforming them into socio-economic independent populace. These transformed beings have the ability which can motivate self and others to become employers of labour and positive contributors to the societies in the scale up of the Gross Domestic Products (GDPs) hence the Gross National Income (GNIs) and the per capita income.

Based on the foregoing, we have a lot at hand. We must rid the streets of the professional beggars though handicapped. Also, the operation 'empower the disabled is total'. Therefore, there is the inevitable need for the empowerment of the physically handicapped citizens, regardless of the gender, age, status, educational attainment, social affiliations and interests in accordance with international best practice. The book shall espouse how the physically challenged can borrow leaf from the saner climes where the physically challenged citizens are employers of labour and wealth creators- **November 10th, 2018**.

<u>**TABLE OF CONTENT**</u>

CHAPTER ONE

<u>INTRODUCTION</u>

All human, regardless of gender, age, race, social esteem, affiliation, is an asset to the wellbeing of the nation and the worlds vice versa. It is a matter of choice of any nation and its stakeholders how they can rally round those born with disabilities and those who are anticipated to living in the condition from being public nuisance or social miscreants but public human assets. As earlier mentioned, the number of people who are becoming disabled every day from the avoidable accidents and preventable epidemics outweighs the number of persons born with disabilities in a proportion of 99% to 1%. If we use the National Bureau of Statistics reports on depression from those causes that would be listed later, we have one out of every five that are suffering from depression and 28% living with chronic depression as at 2016 critically analyzed studies. If the persons are unable to manage the depression, it could lead to disability and decline of the national productivity.

In retrospect, there is no nation without the human beings that populace the geographical area that does not have a challenge or the other. The challenges may not be associated with opulence or indigence but the quality of the states of minds. Failure to manage disappointments, losses, popularity, curtail crises by preventing them, failure to have helping hands and supports, stigmatization, inability to earn living wage, failure to have choices of jobs, spouses, betrayal of close and distant friends, trusted kinsmen and close subordinate, suffering from protracted illnesses that almost defy cure, childlessness after years of marriage, unfaithful spouse, battery husband, night crooning spouse, unsatisfactory relationship among several others are roads to depression which could push abled persons into consumption of non-prescribed drugs or engage in overdosing, driving carelessly and the deadly activities that would lead to the maiming of the limbs and the loss of senses from brains damage. There are people who are celebrities that are not happy with life. There are comedians that crack jokes to make people happy at shows that are not happy within the four corners of their rooms. Many things are not clear to them. Many are afraid of what become of the wealth they have acquired after their death. Many may have problems with their present high ranking as they envisage what happen to the popularity when another person becomes the rave of the moment and the popularity of his faded off. The types of opulence life of their spouses and children may be the reasons for the unhappiness of the persons. By these thoughts running in their minds, they become depressed. Through **depression**, they could engage in drunk driven, engage in illicit sexual activities and living false lives which could lead to injuries to the body or the brains in mental disorder. Without doubt, there is nexus between being disabled and depression. And depression is a product of situations and events on individuals and the environments where they inhabit. The environment people live therefore influences the habits and attitudes to self, families, relatives, neighbours, other people from other ethno-religion circles and the environment by responsibilities and the eventual outputs to the nation and the world in general. People like to be addressed properly and with respect in all societies. The dwarf likes to be addressed like the giant to hold him in high esteem and not as a lowly creature. Every being likes to create storm and be called with great names. Except in some races that do not care about how you address them, a cripple does not desire to be called a cripple. Calling a blind the blind is demeaning to the person and personality. The population of a nation does not exclude the people living with disabilities. With this in mind, the demographic facts and figures at different periods covered all the citizens particularly the citizens. National constitution does not discriminate against any citizen for his or her disability in its Acts. The only lacuna in the constitution is the failure to adequately address the social, economic and political roles of the person with special needs as a result of their disability, inborn or artificial, by amended Acts of legislation.

The human race, able and disabled, could be of one ethnic group and many ethnic descents that meet to live in a place. The ethnic groups have diverse culture and values that promote begging of able and disabled people or not. Some ethnic values hate begging as a trade. Some do not see anything wrong in begging for alms. Human dignity does not count for many of the beggars who do not mind begging within the community people who are close to them are co-habiting. Some out of shame travel to distance places to beg for alms. We have seen people who travelled from the agrarian community in Ibadan to Lagos or Abuja to beg for stipends as alms. People under the guise of performing religion pilgrimage travel to the holy places to collect alms even though they are not living with any disability. What would come to the minds of the disabled who have been abandoned to their fate by the abject stricken society where they live? What moral lesson is got from the able body that travels to distance under any guise to seek for alms to the jobless disabled within?

Nevertheless, begging for alms or financial supports do not mean degrading one's status on the condition and cultural environment such beggars are found. There are cultural environment that are religious but prefer to give out alms to the people living with disabilities instead of empowering them. The givers believe that empowerment of the physically challenged is pushing them hard and a burden to work for their sustenance. *'It is righteous to give alms to those who beg'* many pious said. *'Being disabled is a burden that may not allow the victims to be creative and active on their chosen job'* some admitted. The issue at hand is '<u>does disability mean inability? Does disability connote such disabled cannot be empowered with tools to work with and earn from his or her inputs? Is disability a license to beg for sustenance? Are there no jobs for the people living with disability? Are these persons second citizens as a result of their disabilities?</u> It is appalling to see able-body people that have joined the bandwagon of the beggars line up in the streets begging for alms from the passers-by. Ask those who are not having any body defect the reason for begging for feeding or other basic needs. Many say *'I am unemployed and cannot steal to eat'*. Many liars among would shamelessly say *'I am begging to raise fund for a close relation or family members for the huge medical bills'*. Some feign being fire or motor accident victims. Among those who are physically challenged are those who would hang such inscriptions like *'I am deaf and dumb, help me'*; *'I am blind, help me'*. These inscriptions are underestimating, denigrating and dehumanizing in some cultural environments even though no one raise eyebrow in another. As the economy is biting harder, new methods of begging are launched out. The method of begging and the personality of the 'beggars' shall speak volume about the intention and the interest. There are corporate beggars who are not physically handicapped that have joined the bandwagon of the beggars with body defects.

Millions of the people living with certain physical challenges are born with all the parts of the body intact. But, if the challenge man has in his later life from the negligent of the parents, ignorance in parenting, bad peer group influence and others is a basis of defining a disable, we are all disable simply because everyone is having one challenge or the other. We are not equally gifted and this is the reason for having different types of personalities. There are slow and fast learners. There are slow and fast actors. The bones are stronger than the other. All these natural endowments are never the same aside the artificial causes of disability or disabilities.

Through series of self-inflicts either from ignorance or intentionally, man-caused epidemics from the poor use of the environment leading to toxic pollution of air, water and soil, consumption of poison, the use of deadly and consumption unwholesome of adulterated items, natural disasters such as flood, landslide, earth tremor or earthquake, road accidents, air crash, fire incidents, negligence and incompetent pedtriacs handling baby delivery, attacks, victims of wickedness of man to man like an instance where landmines are planted in the war zones or insecurity volatile areas, heartless revenges by rival ethnic groups, and complicated health challenges, people become maim or loss certain parts of their body. The defects on the body turn them into physically challenged in the society. Those who are lucky to have acquired assets before the incidents may pick up their lives after the incidents and move on with lives. The dependents at the period such strange illness or accidents occur may lose hope especially if the trauma experts are not involved to put them back to the right path. There are misfortunes from the crops of bad leadership leading to malnourish of the vulnerable people which could lead to their physical disability. The insecurity from attacks from the gangs, terrorists and the bandits or gunmen from different sources could result into the maiming of people. We have read many disabled people that were caught up between the rival militant or rebel groups' crossfire or intentional dismembering of the parts of their body. Sierra Leoneans and migrant Africans would never forget the criminalities of the rebels that cut hands and legs of the innocent people, especially aliens cut in the crossfire from hostile nations to their cause, regardless of their gender and age by the hard-drugged and intoxicated militants. In the workplaces, many employers of labour do not see the safety kits as a primary provision to avoid accidents in the premises. Many people living with disabilities are from the avoidable injuries sustained in the course of doing their duties at the ill-equipped workplaces. Unfortunately, such companies or employers do not have insurance covers for their workers after failing to put in places the safety kits for the workers. Structural defects in the building of the companies could cost lives and asset during inferno. What is expected from a factory with only one exit in a case of fire incident? What about a factory without fire extinguishers? Would the workers in factory be able to escape from the inferno in such badly constructed work environment? On the part of the nations, failure to budget for the people living with disabilities by the government of the nation add fuels to the fire as the victims turn themselves into beggars to survive. Truly speaking, nation used to have adequately funded special homes for special people who are born with the physical challenges. There are schools for the deaf and dumb, schools for the blinds, schools for the cripples even the mentally disorder patients in psychiatric hospitals. The lesser the funding of the institutions by the government, the lesser the treatment of the people living with disabilities and the more the economic burden on their relatives and families! As the economic situation, micro and macro, decline and worsen generally especially in the period of economic recession, the families and relatives who have also become financially handicapped abandoned them to their fates. By this, the handicaps who are not trained to work with the limbs or the available resources within their reach have to be on the streets begging for survival.

Along the streets in the poor nation especially those who claimed to be religious are beggars. Most of these beggars are crippled, blind, leper or with one disability or the other. There are also destitute who feign disability by the physical outlooks. One thing that comes to my mind *'are they incapable of working and creating wealth with the nature of disability?* By studies of the wealthy disabled in the other nations especially in Europe, these are right examples and models who are not disable by productivity to the national output even though they are physically challenged. The standpoint remained that 'disabilities are not disabilities in outputs. All living souls have potentials from natural endowments despite some physical challenges. If someone has no eyes to read, there are braille courses for reading. Someone who can read could be able to write to trouble shoot the challenges read in prints. Someone who is lame could apply their senses to engage themselves positively. Such could be orators, motivational speakers, stand-up comedian, readers, poets, and author of books. They could be thespians in films and documentaries. The society such lives help him or her the more to build careers of choice.

The mission to eliminate beggars from our streets is inevitable to all stakeholders. To achieve this, everyone has role to play. The focus is on how the beggars who are truly handicapped can be positively empowered and motivated spiritually to be financially and economically independent. People can launch to seek for funds for certain classes of people especially the vulnerable, the widow, widowers, the orphans, the specially challenged and the sick who can barely feed not to talk of paying for the medical services and drugs. In this work, our focus is on the people who are truly challenged physically and helpless in the midst of harsh economy.

Being born as disable is not a disease or ridicule. Being a disable by accident is not demeaning. Man is what he thinks he is. In the world of today are those born with disabilities that are leaders and mentors of crowds of able body. In the history of Shonghai Empire, the cripple boy, **Sundiata**, was the conqueror of the Sumangurus of Susu Empire. In the history of the religion of Islam was **Abdullahi bin Maktum**, a blind but learned and pious in Islamic precepts, that became a governor under a caliph. All individuals are naturally endowed with knowledge, skill and talent or the others waiting to be optimally explored for the glory and advancement of mankind. Looking at the fancy and exotic structures in the nations of the world, many are owned by the people living with disabilities. Many a business that is thriving is owned by the disabled persons. There are inventions from the brains of intelligent and brilliant disabled in history. The challenges facing some disabled people especially those with amputated limbs that are replaced by artificial limbs, the persons living with blind sight that are reading with braille technology and the likes pave the way for the innovations and the inventions. It is only those whose brains have been diseased that can be said to be non-productive among the disabled. The world has produced several wealthy people among the people living with disabilities. Some are not born with any disability but are later become victims of accidents to have the defect of the body. A man with active limbs and senses today could become defective by sickness, accidents, incidents and such tomorrow. The motto in the minds of everyone is that disability in never an inability. A way starts where a way ends. They can be disabled but are rich in ideas and thoughts. All of them have viable business ideas that have employed millions worldwide. **John Foppe** is armless but a renowned motivational speaker earning big from motivating people into higher productivity. **Walt Disney** had a net worth of $5 billion as an American film producer, director, screenwriter, voice actor, animator, entrepreneur, entertainer and international philanthropist. He was a co-founder of Walt Disney Productions that is worth $35 billion, best known motion picture producers in the world. **Stevie Wonder** is an American musician, composer, multi-instrumentalist, singer and songwriter who started his career at the age of eleven from Motown records. By estimated value, he is worth $110 million. The world would never be complete without the mentioning the successful author, actor, producer and activist in **Michael J. Fox** whose net-worth is $65 million despite his disability. In Nigeria, **Chinualumogu Albert Achebe** (1930-2013) was healthy living professor and author of several bestselling books till 1990 when he had a fatal accident in Nigeria. Through the accident, he was paralysed from the waist to the legs. Despite this challenge at the period of life, he taught at Bard College at New York between 1991 and 2009. He won Man Booker International Prize Award in 2007. In 2012, he released the popular and bestseller book 'There was a country: a personal history of Biafra'. Also, the popular singer like the late **Dan Maraya** of Jos was influential and rich from songs despite his impaired sight. **Evangelist Doctor Olayinka Joel Ayefele**was born without any body defect in Ipoti Ekiti in Ekiti state of Nigeria. He was a renowned broadcaster, jingle producer, on air personality, fast rising star and migrating fast towards becoming a veteran in communication media business before he had an accident in the course of his duty. He eventually started his business empire after the accident that befell him in the 90's starting with the release a chartbuster album titled 'Bitter Experience'. He is worth billions of naira by the estimated values of his Fresh FM radio communication businesses in the southwest states and other businesses outside the shores of the nation today. Despite his position, he is a popular and creative gospel singer, entertainer, seasoned broadcaster, celebrity, socialite, entrepreneur, multi-instrumentalist, and a renowned philanthropist. One of the popular Grand Khadis, a revered Islamic cleric, chief Imam, author of Islamic books, role model, mentor, philanthropist, Islamic scholar that had issued a lot of fatwas was **Sheikh ibn Bas** in Saudi Arabia who had visual challenge. **Prophet Timothy Obadare**, Of CAC WOSEM, was renowned evangelist, highly celebrated, role model priest, emeritus pastor in the southwest Nigeria and the world despite his disability. **Prophet Moses Muideen kasali,** not born blind according to him, is a counsellor, mentor, model, socialite, philanthropist and preacher of the gospel known across the world. In the history of the broadcasting media industry, the popular on the air personality broadcasting on wheelchair, **Bolanle Kareem** of the then Ogun state broadcasting corporation was physically challenged. **Oscar Pistorius** was a popular award winning athlete in South Africa running short distances to the podium with artificial legs. In different physically challenged sports, there are record makers and breakers from the competitions especially those organized at the advanced nations. All of the successful personalities have impacted the world of mankind with their wealth of natural resources which the business environment has provided from different shades, sizes and shapes of supports. A moral lesson from the great personalities identified show that there is no limit to the target achievement for all regardless of the type of physical disability.

In the light of the above, no one living with disability should give up hope and resigned to begging for survival. The successful entrepreneurs among those born with disabilities and those who suffer disabilities at the latter part of their lives are able to manage their crises to be something out of nothing. They effectively manage their depression within and outside their inner chambers. They live with the positive spirits to have these positive and motivating thoughts like *'disability is never an inability'*. *'I am not the worst among men. I am better than many others'*. *'I have the most precious in life. I have hope unlike the dead'*. *'If I fail to be hopeful and live a quality life, the life would be a jungle to live'*. *'I have invaluable and unique resources that can make me an asset'. 'If so so person with similar challenge can make it, what stops me?'* among others. Life is full of challenges and is bound to create new challenges. We are all transiting from position to position, grade to grade. Our dreams would never die premature unless we give up striving to hit it in life. Our people living with disabilities have countless mentors and role models in the wealthy people among those that have the physical challenges across the world. Some questions that must run our system are 'if the people living with disabilities can make it to the podium abroad, what is stopping our own people here? Where did we get it wrong to integrate our own people with disability to achieve their dreams? Is physical challenge a natural curse in this part of the world? How are the nations abroad able to tap and harness the resources in the disabled persons to turn them into celebrity and wealthy? On the basis of the posers, the focus should therefore be how to rid the streets of beggars especially among those having one physical challenge or the other and also transform the beggars in to wealth and employment creators from the level of ridicule.

In addition, if the disabled are not properly integrated and absorbed into the society as part of the contributors and human assets, then the number of human liabilities shall grow by the day since men are losing one limb or the other to avoidable accidents on roads, incidents at homes and offices, maladministration of drugs and the misuse of injections by quacks. Steps must be taken to rid the homes, streets and the nations of people living with disabilities. The steps are useful guides to minimize the numerical strength of the people living with disabilities across the nation.

<u>STEPS</u>

Firstly, take a census or the disabled lists of the people living with disabilities by wherever they are found. As anticipated, the number increases by the day especially by the number of amputees who lost their limbs after accidents, self-inflicted issues, spousal battery, attacks and the likes. Sensitize the public to earn support for the census of these people. Publicly and privately preach against stigmatization in order to have the anticipated cooperation from the public and the government. The collaboration efforts between the social welfare ministry or relevant agencies with the non-governmental organization and the religion societies of all denomination shall do the magic.

Secondly, all the preventable measures that could lead into disabilities one is not born with should be identified and prevented. A wise says *'avoid crises is the solution to manage crises'*. If those who are not born with a disability or the other are our focus, we should minimize the exposure to the risks leading to the loss of limbs or the senses which would shore up the number of people living with disabilities. Numerous are what the stakeholders led by the leaders at all levels to eliminate all the risk factors. All hands must be on deck to critically analyse the causes from the reports and studies of records of victims. This studying must know that we are all potential disable from the reckless way of living and consumption. By this in mind, we must be prepared to treat every disable person like ourselves. We must abhor turning into the people living with a disabilities into becoming professional beggars. The people who have taken up begging as a job should be made to hate begging for survival. Begging demeans persons ant their personalities as the beggars are scorn at in the sight of the charity-givers. The physically challenged should not curse the Creator who creates what HE wills and fashions all creatures how HE desires in accordance with the revelations from the incorruptible scriptures.

Thirdly, all the persons living with disabilities should never underestimate themselves; they should always think within and outside the box to proffer solutions to their socio-economic crises with the use of the available resources and facilities at their beck and call. Discover what you are naturally endowed with. Think over what you can use all the senses for. The sense of hearing, sense of seeing, sense of thinking, sense of feeling or perceiving and the likes are at their disposal for unveiling potentials in employments that can be created and worked upon by the physically challenged persons. This is applicable to those who do not have limbs to support movement from places to places.

Fourthly, all the people should make efforts to identify their constitutional rights to seek redress and reviews where and when necessary. The disability clauses must be regularly worked upon. Everyone must know their limits and rights in order to be responsible citizens of high reverence.

Fifthly, there should be cooperation of the stakeholders to produce the persons living with disabilities to the public and gathering where their natural resources could be worked upon by career counselors, psychologists, sociologists, medical care counselors, motivators, mentors, role models and the likes. In such gathering, all the tools for different jobs should be freely distributed after all the supports for them to live quality lives like those who have no defects. By this, the walking tools for the blind and the cripple, the vision or braille material for reading to the blind, the audio tool for the people with hearing issue. The non-governmental organizations, corporate organizations, philanthropists, the religion associations, alumnus or alma mater, voluntary associations or the social clubs should support the government to make available right tools for those living with different challenges.

Sixth, self-motivation is a key. One with a disability should be happy in the condition and never be moody. In the world, there are people living with greater challenges even among the people without any disability. In any condition, they should be happy.

Seventh, the stakeholders in the nation must be on top of their responsibilities by playing their primary roles as and when due in order to avoid creating vacuums which could affect the people living with disabilities. We should see them as our siblings who deserve equal rights. We must incorporate all the people living with disabilities into the societies with no form of discrimination. We must live with them without any prejudice. All the disabled must be on special care and attention more than the others who have the ability to move and seek for help at any time of urgency.

Eighth, respect is reciprocal, we should accord them respect in the private and public engagements. The right and befitting titles should be used while addressing them. Old age related diseases can relegated them to the wheel. They should be rightly recognized in the scheme of things. The proverb should be 'what an able body person can do, the disable can also do the same'. This shall create sense of belonging and push them into high productivity and contribution to the outputs of the nation in general

Ninth, the stakeholders should expose the people to secondary value chains of different sectors that can become sources of income to them. On the part of the people with special needs, they should also grab all opportunities open for the citizens as they are not excluded. If the capable work in the farm, the farm produce can be packaged and sold by the people with disabilities provided the right environment for this to happen has been created. In order to increase the knowledge and interests, certain provisions must be made. Such provisions include free and compulsory education, scholarship, grants, bursary, loans and free workshops to boost their inborn talents, skills and other human capacity.

Tenth, all stakeholders, starting from the families and the communities including the public places specially designed for the physically challenged, should accord them respect and tolerate their possible excesses. All forms of depression should be preventable by proffering practicable solutions at the right time before it is too late. None should live with depression by the opening of the depressive treated centres in all communities, offices, establishments, institutions and organizations. Mothers-to-be must be prepared for the babies by strictly observe all the pre-natal and post natal care for the fetus and the baby. There should be no room for self-medication during the pregnancy. Right diets should be consumed. Right exercise should be done. Healthy environment should be place of habitation. The father should adequately provide for the pregnant mothers with provisions and monitoring, supervising and motivating them to keep observing the doctor's guides in order to be delivered of sound and healthy baby. If the baby is delivered with a deformity, special care must be given by the parents based on the doctor's guide. Parents should not be stigmatized against children born with defects. Treat them first before your turn. Give them the first class treatment in order to prevent thinking of being second class citizens. The community should also observe equality in the treatment of the special children. Government and associations should crown the efforts of the parents and the residents in the proper care of the children living with disabilities.

N.B. All the steps are in not in order as they could rearrange by the discretion of the readers and stakeholders. Aside the care for the persons living with disabilities at our vicinity by the references, we must avoid the artificial causes of disabilities especially depression.

CHAPTER TWO

<u>WHO ARE DISABLED?</u>

As aforementioned, the Nigerian constitution does not define a citizen called 'disabled'. By the word 'citizen' or 'citizens' in the constitution, it comprises all the natives born, registered and unregistered, of diverse ethnic groups and faiths in the geographic entity within the landmass of over 923,000 square kilometer. In short, citizenry is not defined as those who are physically strong and sound senses. But, by parental and professional negligence including the leadership failure, citizens could become disabled. Man is expected to be born with all the limbs and senses intact. There is no denial to the fact that some, very minute in number compared to those who become disabled later in life, are born with body defects especially at the pre-natal and post natal care periods. Deadly mistakes by negligence of the delivery workers are wrongly attributed to natural defects. The defects could be detected early or in the later years after birth. External factors could instigate the causes of disabilities. The misuse of skin costumes like the cancerous bleaching creams and soap, badly preserved with contaminated preservatives could lead to disabilities in the consumers. Age-long traditions that are injurious such as tribal marks and circumcision of the female genitals could lead to one disability or the other. We can therefore identify the <u>first category</u> to be those who have **PHYSICAL CHALLENGES** as the disable. By this, the disabled are simply the people living with disabilities who are either born with the disabilities or as a result of accidents, epidemics, frustrations, depression or other unmanageable incidents. Such could be blind, cripple, deaf and dumb naturally by birth or by accidents from self-inflict or external factors.

The <u>second category</u> is those who have **MENTAL DISORDER** which could be traced to such ailments like depression, low esteem and the likes. The disorder could also be self-inflict or by spiritual attacks by studies. None is free from depressive tendencies leading to become disabled. Man needs to have enough courage to identify the signs of depression, frustrations, disappointments, losses, failures in order to be able to manage self from all the identifiable causes of disabilities by observing 'the avoids', do's and don'ts in order to live quality life that would not endanger the limbs and the brains contained in the book from the author titled **"Zero Depression"**. Several issues could also lead to any of the causes as published in the recommended book from the stable of the author. Such could be diseases with terminal ailments that keep recurring without healing despite all the curative measures from the specialists. Such could also be suffering from malnourish as a result of famine from long years of drought leading to food shortage in supplies, insecurity, displacement, kidnapping or victims of human traffickers. By the two, there are persons that stammer or talk senselessly as a result. Many have the skins burnt and facial burn by the use of contaminated bleaching creams and soaps. When man becomes hater of self as a result of the negative reactions of self or quack-prescribed drugs, creams, soaps, diets and the likes, this is a disability from the mindset as such feels inferior to the others. This could make him or her to misbehave abnormally. Having looked into different ways people could become disabled, we have to encourage the nation and the stakeholders on how to transform them from being human liabilities into human assets.

The third category is those who are victims of crises such as insecurity, wars and economic sanctions. Many who are born with all the limbs intact could become disenable to add right outputs in size to the GDP with the shortage of basic needs at their beck and call. These produce destitute who flood the streets since they are homeless and survive by mercy of God through the charity-givers. All the kinds of disabilities are not right licenses to become human burdens on others and the nation. Every man has natural gifted to break out of their shells to retain their integrity and dignity as human assets.

In summary, there are defects that can be corrected through relevant surgery, professional counseling and the use of relevant devices. It is a responsible of the parents, the communities, the philanthropic organizations, the associations, the institutions, the employers and the nation, who are stakeholders, to take the right steps to search for medical attention to have solutions on the defective part. There are specialized hospitals for the babies and children born with disabilities. Even, the accident victims who lost limbs could have artificial limbs at the hospitals. By these, no one with a disability should resign their fate to living till death with the disability in this century with advanced knowledge. What can we infer? It is simply said that *'disability is a thing of the mind just as age is a count of years'*. If the wealthy people who are disabled in the other worlds had lost hope by their disabilities, they would find it impossible to harness their potentials to the fullest. The situations and the prevalent environment may not be hindrances to set up a target. The wealthy disabled in the part of the world see themselves as capable as the able body people.

By tradition, some primitive customs and beliefs could lead to the disability. Certain training and the environments where the trainings are taken place could also pave the way to one form of disability or the other.

Generally, the largest percentage of new births, in population, is not disabled but each birth is naturally gifted. Many aged could be free from paralysis if right medical care is given. The only visible exception is the conjoined twins. This is a challenge that is natural. All other forms of disabilities could be traced to self-infliction and corruption which occur early or later in the life of man.

SUMMARIZED CAUSES OF DISABILITY

The categories of disabilities are two namely natural and artificial-based. We can further expand the causes or factors leading to disabilities into the following:

a) **SELF-INFLICT:** This is multifaceted and countless variable from person to person, from region to region and environment to environment. It has to do with all causes of depression and loss of personal discipline and failure to comply with simple rules. Introverts are closer to become depressed and these depressive disorders could lead to self-injuries resulting into the paralyses of the body. Failure to play one's civic responsibilities is also a path to depression. Failure to correct one's bad attitudes to life makes life a place not worthy to live and hence leads to depression that can cause disabilities. By this, the level of popularity, the exotic houses being lived, the custom built cars at the garage and the luxuries being enjoyed do not make life worthy to many and therefore immerse in depression that could lead to attempts to end one's life or the destruction of other's lives. Rejections of pregnancies by the 'husbands' especially when the babies are the products of extra marital sexual relationship could turn the mothers into depression. Failure of the husbands to lovingly support the dutiful mothers and the children could push the women and children or the household into depression. Imitation of another person could lead to unnecessary and dangerous rivalry. All these are gateway to increase the number of persons living with disabilities from self-inflict actions. Depressed medical practitioners could administer wrong injections that would cripple the sick. Depressed drivers could drive recklessly to kill or maim self and other road users. People could get paralyses from the bad consumables. Someone who drinks intoxicants has invited ailments like cirrhosis, and if such hits his head on the bare ground, epilepsy could sneak in to the body leading to the cripple of the limbs from stroke. The consumption of cheap unwholesome drugs or the patronage of fake medical physicians could lead to paralysis of the body or the paralysis or the 'dead' of the brains. Many have been rendered handicapped from the misuse of the electronic devices such as high decibels that can deafen the ear faculty, the exposure of the eyes to the rays from the tubes without protection of the eyes. Individuals should be wary of what they consume in foods, beverages, drugs and the likes; they should be mindful of the environment they live as man should live in water-borne, air-born and harsh weather conditions to have quality living. The persons that have deformity should not imitate the physically strong fellows in the public places to avoid aggravating the disabilities. The manner of handling objects should be done according to the instructions and the directives of the producers in order to prevent injuries that could lead to disabilities. Those who overstep boundary of consuming expired products and contaminated foods and drinks have attracted ailments that can open the room for disabilities. People who fail to consult the specialized physicians when symptoms are noticed are liable to become a disable. The earlier the right professional and consultant is contacted, the earlier the ills have been nipped in the buds. By shared stories, many have become paralyzed for the ignorance use of electronic items. The misuse of mobile phones at the cooking room or kitchens, switch on of the phone at the places of electricity generating set which could ring at the time of putting on the generator, the non-challant attitude like smoking of cigarettes at fuel stations or at the time of dispensing the premium motor spirit to the vehicle, the misuse of sharp tools that can harm the bodies could injure the body of those handling them, careless driving or over speeding along the road, overloading of vehicles leading to the burst of tyre and fatal accidents on the highways among several self-inflict causes. The frequent use of quack health workers could result into the administration of deadly injections. In some cases, low esteem and depression could push people into committing crimes against self which can result into disability. Inability to manage matrimonial crises could push man into injuring oneself. We have seen ladies and gents whose bad driving from bad emotion has resulted into fatal accidents that claimed part of the limbs. Many who have lived a submissive life would understand how to live a happy life no matter the conditions, favourable or unfavourable. On the last note, anybody that could not effectively and efficiently manage personal crises with anticipated approaches would enter into depression and liable to become disabled. Ask me the solution over frustrations, disappointments, deprivations, denials and the countless shapes and sizes leading to depressive state is solved if one can be submissive and use the opposite to solve the crises. Submissiveness means observe the prescriptions and the proscriptions of God. Secondly, get a right replacement in either complementary or substitute. If a wife divorced you, get another spouse. If a job is lost, search for another. If your employer does not promote you, seek another workplace. If rising inflation has eaten your disposal income, create additional sources of income or reduce your consumption. In short, for all ailments are solutions or the cure so reported from the lips of the noblest to guide mankind.

b) **INORDINATE AMBITION:** The human lusts for the acquisition of material wealth, ranking in positions of authority, rivalry for economic gains in the amassing of wealth such as fleet of exotic and customized cars, mansions at highbrow and government reservation areas, occupying the exalted position in the public, rivalry over the control and marriage to beautiful damsels and the likes are pushing into competitive races. Studies show that many are involving in accidents more at the tail ends of the year as a result of the ambition to meet the targets in assets before the year runs out. By this, the numbers of the disabled like amputees, those who lost their sight to disconnection of nerves of the eyes or dislocations, loss of memory via shocks during accidents and the likes increase. Many could have spiritual attacks from the rituals for money leading to insanity or greater depression.

c) **FACTORY-INFLICT:** Safety tools that are not provided by the employers could result in the maiming of the employees. Failure to equip the work premises with fire extinguishers could result into destroyer of assets and maim lives. There should be right sanctions and stiff punitive measures against the establishments that do not install the relevant security and safety facilities at the workplaces for the protection of the management, workers and visitors.

d) **GOVERNMENT IRRESPONSIBILITY:** The nation that fails in its responsibility to build right social infrastructures has exposed the citizens into insecurity in different forms and sizes. Government is expected to empower the marriage act to make provision for all marital issues that can lead to separation or divorce and distant marriage which may not allow the lovely bond between the man and the wife with their children. Parenting should be critically addressed in the Marriage Act. Administration fails to inject adequate resources in capital to education not to talk of declaring free and qualitative education for all regardless of the ability and the disabilities. What about the efforts of the government to reduce the cost of living for every citizen to be able to afford all the basic needs? As a result of failure in leadership, crimes escalate on daily basis. Preventable epidemics are spreading like viral. There are series of avoidable accidents every day. People have accidents on the potholed roads to sustain injuries that could lead to the amputation of limbs. The amputees that do not have a legitimate source of living before the accidents could prefer to beg along the streets instead of involving all the crimes like stealing, armed robbery, vandalization, products fakery, frauds, kidnapping for ransom and other crimes.

e) **INSECURITIES:** Racial and religion crises could lead to physical and mental disabilities from attacks from different rivalry groups. Hatred of races and the animosity against the adherents of opposing faiths could trigger deadly violence and orchestrated attacks that can render people crippled or disabled.

f) **HEALTH HAZARDS:** The environmental challenges from the misuse of the environment especially from the pollution lead to the hazard to the people. Avoid contaminated water, soil and air. Never consume contaminated foods and drugs. Do not use expired tyres for your vehicle. Drive with caution by obeying the traffic and driving rules.

g) **EPIDEMICS:** The poor use of environmental resources like water, the land and the air is a pathway to diseases. The water-borne and air-borne diseases are some of the causes of the disabilities in the victims. The six child-killer diseases have been attributed to the causes of ailments that affect the people negatively. Many children are disabled from the child-killer diseases if they are not properly taken care of.

h) **STRANGE ILLNESS:** People could be affected by spiritual attacks leading to the maiming of the body. In some cases, the poor use of the environment especially the land, water and air pollution leading to airborne and water borne diseases often leads to 'strange diseases'. The medical researches categorize the viruses that are not known in the disease research history as 'strange'. The monkey pox, the ebola virus, the sexual transmitted diseases and the likes could be the basis for strange illnesses. In the years back, small pox had killed several children before the vaccination was developed. The lassa fever and the ebola virus in some parts of central Africa, if not properly attacked and cured, could end in the paralysis of the body if the victims do not lose their lives. The consumption of diseased or wild animals and birds could result into illnesses that may defy cure and therefore open ways for disabilities. Avoid the spread of epidemics. Treat the water, soil and air especially when contaminated before use.

i) **DRUG ABUSE:** This does not limit to the indigent but the opulent and the celebrities who seek drugs such as antidepressants to end some causes of depression. They live on drug to kill depressive ailments to no avail and the adverse effect of drug consumption is open way to disability. Many do not know that depression is not curable by drugs but attitudes (Reference: "**Zero Depression**"). The violation of the prescriptions by the pharmacists could lead to abnormal growth of the limbs. Today, all the banned drugs are being consumed by youths resulting into their loss of memory, limbs and treatment strange diseases which are adverse effects of the drugs that have been abused. This is as a result of self-medication and the excessive use of drugs through overdosing. In some cases, the failure or refusal to abide by the instructions from the pharmacists that drugs should be kept away from the reach of the children could lead to self-destruct.

j) **POOR PARENTING:** Generation must not fail the next generation by the failure in parenting responsibility. No man and wife should abandon their individual responsibility not to talk of transferring the burdens on each other when both are capable, morally and financially, to effectively and efficiently execute the responsibilities. The dissolve of marriage and the abandon of responsibility should not be under the guise of loss sources of finance. Parents must find alternative sources of earning legitimately to fulfill their financial obligations over the children. The issue of illegal marriage that could produce illegitimate children should be a thing of the past by laws and traditions. No baby should be abandoned to a parent as a result of having a disability. And there should be no room for part time or trial couple to avoid running away from one's parental responsibilities. Parents whose sexual intercourse produces a baby or babies (in twins, triplets, quadruple and more) should be ready to parent. They should mould the character of the child through right trainings from age one to be right personality in life. Introvert and extrovert are products from bad parenting at homes. Life requires living in moderation to avoid the excesses opening to disability. Many who are born with the perfect conditions at birth become maimed by the neglect of the parents especially the mothers. There are abandoned babies as a result of poverty especially by the professional prostitutes who have no room for settling down with any man in marriage.

k) **INEXPERIENCED AND INCOMPETENT HEALTH WORKER:** By complaints, many who are healthy are rendered disabled from the unsterilized syringes, wrong drug administration and wrong injections of the inexperienced and incompetent doctors or nurses attending to the patients at wards. Health workers particularly the pediatrics should undergo periodical trainings, on and off the job, on how to handle baby and child care in a way that no harm shall be inflicted on them from pregnancy till birth. Many suffering from diabetes and other diseases walk or drive themselves to the hospitals only to come out as amputees as a result of wrong dosage, toxic injection and neglect by the ill-motivated and incompetent medical staff attending to them. Many of the medical team have forgotten the ethic codes and pledge of the health service job to save and protect lives.

l) **UNWANTED PREGNANCIES AND ABORTION:** In the course of aborting the unwanted pregnancies, victims could damage any inner organs which would lead to the deformity of the parts of the body. Many of the fetus have become infected from the wombs of the mothers-to-be as a result of the intoxicants and drug abuse during the trimesters of the pregnancies.

m) **YOUTHFUL EXUBERANCE:** As a result of the feeling of sense of belonging to the youth circles, many youths embrace bad gangs to claim self-glory and command undeserved respects. The joining of gangs that drink intoxicants to stupor, sniffing of hard drugs and the dangerous driving under influence of drugs could lead to self-inflict injuries. Gangs fight dangerously with dangerous weapons on flimsy reasons and insignificant issues such as over ladies, control of the street. Many youths celebrate their birthdays and other ceremonies with intoxicants, over-speed while on the wheels, and never respect the roads signs.

n) **NATURAL DISASTERS:** Except it is a test from God and the test should be for a purpose, natural disaster could be traced to the poor use of the environment by man. The climate change and its adverse effects are from the misuse of the environmental resources and failure to keep tidy the resources. If the world decides to live in aesthetic environment and team up in sensitizing the nations on how keep the water, atmosphere and land clean, and afforestation is encouraged just as evacuation and recycling of wastes are done by all the nations, there would not be all the spiral effects of climate changes. Nations would harvest resources in the water, forests, air and lands bountifully to grow their economies. People would have enough to feed themselves as water would be adequate for all purposes, domestic, recreation and industrial. There would not be epidemics, unemployment and all other factors leading to depression shall be reduced to the insignificant minimum. And the incidence of people being becoming disabled shall be reduced to almost zero.

In summary, we have emphasized that depression is adding majorly to the increasing number of persons living with disabilities. Aside the self-inflict, we look at what other forms of depressive disorders are having on the PLWDs. Let us share some of these by showing the causes and the aftermath on the people.

a) **FAILURES:** It has to do with the result of human efforts that do not come into fruition after all relentless inputs and optimism. Failing in examination after putting efforts. Failing in having the right and dream person to marry. Failing to have the right environment to live. Failing to have trusty people around one. Failing to find right job after service with excellent result. Failing to earn profits after sales. Failure to achieve a goal, failure to have the desire basic needs which may come from violations, cheating and denials. Everyone desires to be successful in his chosen career. He wants to be first in class as student, desires to win the prize for excellence, to snatch the sole ticket in a race, politics, to have the best of material wealth, to control the largest in resources, to be the cynosure of all eyes, to be at the top position as boss

b) **DEPRIVATIONS:** Every person can be deprived of one thing or the other leading to the depression of the deprived. Boss can deprive the subordinates their dues. Masters can deprive the messengers their due rights to extend depression to them through disappointments. Government can create depression in people when a trusted administration fails to religiously observe the primary responsibilities to impact the lives of the citizens positively but instead engage in massive looting of the treasury. Many a couple become depressed when they lost their loved ones, when they could have satisfactory sexual relationship, when there is sudden divorce paper filed at court, when one of them packed out of the matrimonial homes over trivial issue, when the husband or wife catches one another red handed playing extra marital affair especially on their matrimonial bed, when their highly trusted and loved spouses cheat on them, when they cannot make adequate provision for their family members from the lean source of income, when they have rights abused by the oppressive neighbours, when the community they reside is trampling on their human right, when their children are not growing, brilliant at academics or join gangs and behaving like miscreants. If they could not find peace and happiness within the homes, the office duties would suffer and this emotional challenge shall be transferred to their clients at work. A doctor husband may administer wrong injections to the sick which would paralyse the body hence turns the sick into disable.

c) **RIGHTS ABUSE:** A situation where the rules and regulations are not duly observed opens the way for abuses in different forms. This could push people into doing negative things not minding the adverse effects on the body and the other persons around and beyond. If a motorist abuses the right of the other road users, accidents are caused and people are injured leading to amputation of any of the limbs, loss of eye sight and brain damage. We have seen situations where drivers drive contrary to the road regulation and therefore over speed against the speed limit to kill or maim many innocent passers-by on the pedestrians. One can imagine the number of the rights abuses that have led to the paralyses people suffer on daily basis.

d) **LACK OF MOTIVATION:** Every worker deserves right motivation as and when due to be excellent in the course of their duties. They require right incentives in a right work environment with right remuneration to be outstanding in performance. Failure to pay workers right wage called living wage but slave wage would demoralize them and hence their inputs in the works would never be something to write home about. All social service workers that are deprived of right tools and welfare package would never raise their productivity. And this shall have spiral adverse effects on the people they work with and on.

e) **BAD ROLE MODELS AND MENTORS:** People imitate revered people to be active and reference point. They see them as mirrors and as people with exemplary character. If those they highly revered fail to match their talks with walks, then they have become bad models and reverence to others. The frustrations from the parallel behavior of the models and mentors would not bring positive thoughts to the minds of the people who previously adore them. Let us give some instances. A doctor that admonished the psychiatric patient not to smoke marijuana must not smoke same. If such doctor is caught smoking marijuana, then that is the end of the talk. No patient suffering from the ailment would take him serious again. A marriage counselor that advised the couple to avoid extra marital affair would lose his or her respect the moment he or she is caught red handed in extra marital affairs. If the couples play the outside match and got infected, the infection could lead to the loss of any part of the body and therefore rendered such disabled.

<u>ARE THEY REALLY DISABLED?</u>

Disability is a thing of the mind though could be physical noticed if someone has body defects or such abnormality is shown during interactions testing the sense of feeling, seeing, speaking, hearing and thinking. Generally, people are living with one form of disability or the other by inborn feature, child-birth complications and the accidental discharge later in life from avoidable incidents. Yet, from the previous discussion definition of who a disable is in the society, we have established the fact that every man that lacks certain features of a complete person is a disable. We mean an incomplete person by physical features and not necessary by the material (assets), mental and spiritual resources. We are talking about a physical feature which includes Impaired or bad eyesight sight through glaucoma, cataract and other eye diseases, slur speech or stammering, inability to hear, inability to cripple and the likes are signs of disability. Some are slow learners as a result of dull brains or natural intelligence. The people who suffer from autism and Down Syndrome could be categorized as some of those living with physical disabilities. They are not disabled by intellectual property, by the degree of thinking faculty and what they can do with their limbs, from the natural endowments. Being a cripple does not mean that the person cannot be at the top of their jobs provided they can put into use the natural abilities. The histories of the wealthy people living with physical disabilities in the world are a confirmation that disability is never an inability. They are capable of converting what they have to wealth of resources.

In retrospect, there is the need for instilling confidence in the people living with a deformity or the other. Just as the age is a thing of number and of the mind, being disabled should be seen as the thing that is irrelevant. Disability is therefore a thing of the mind. Those who are truly physically handicapped in the saner climes are capable and creative in mind. A dwarf should never see self as dwarf but a giant with tall ambition. This should be the mindset of the people living with disabilities in order to harness their full potentials.

<u>RESOURCES AVAILABLE TO THE DISABLED</u>

Like the others, all disabled people have the following at their beck and call:

a) **FUNDAMENTAL HUMAN RIGHT:** All creatures have rights not to talk of human beings regardless of their body defects. The national constitutions identify persons living with disability as part and parcel of the nation with all the rights to live a quality life, right to life, right to live in aesthetic environment, right to have access to all that can impact their lives, right to associate and dissociate, right of religion, right to quality education, quality health care services, effective and efficient transportation, quality security or protection, free movement and several other rights combined to have equality, justice and fairness. With these, they can dream and set the ball rolling to have their dreams come true with all supports from the nation and the other stakeholders.

b) **FACULTIES:** Most who are not having disease like dementia can apply the other senses that are sound to identify potentials. Those who have eyes and hand without legs can venture into clerical jobs in the public and private sectors. By the senses, many are brilliantly creative to contribute to the outputs in the nation.

c) **TIME RESOURCES:** The time is at their disposal to learn new skills from listening to news, messages and information. They should create time to read books. Joining the book reading club to share ideas would assist them to starting viable business ideas.

d) **COMMUNITY EMPATHY:** By studies, people patronize the products and services of the people than those that have the ability to move distance to locate their customers.

e) **FREEBIES:** Through the love for the persons living with disabilities, donations come from different corners to improve the financial empowerment towards boosting their economic powers.

f) **INDEPENDENCE:** They are independent to be masters of themselves unless they decide to lower their social esteem through begging to sustain themselves. No citizen is inferior to another. We have equal opportunities to aspire to become a public figure, acquire wealth legitimately, socialize without restriction, freedom of association, religion, marry and procreate.

<u>ENDING SELF-INFLICT PATHS TO DISABILITY</u>

Having established that majority of the people living with disabilities are from human errors before and after births, then there is the need to look at what can be done to reduce to the insignificant minimum the incidence of self-inflict challenges that defect the body. There are steps by the stakeholders to avoid normal persons becoming disabled. Some of these steps to end or scale down self-inflict traced disabilities are:

a) **CONSTITUTIONAL REVIEW:** The administration should uphold the rights enshrined in the constitution to protect the lives of the unborn by the parents and the pedtriacs through Marriage and Baby or Child Right. The right should forbid abandon of any baby or child as a result of his or her disability. The social welfare department should be empowered with incentives and resources to take over the care of the disabled baby or child from the indigent or dead parents. Also, the major cause of disability, depression should be recognized in the law where all the causes and solutions are enshrined in the constitution. By these, the lives and property of the citizens in order pushing the citizens into the state of depression which could open the path to self-destruct with intoxicants and hard drugs. In addition, the constitution should plan for disabled and expand the scope of those who are disabled to include those who are vulnerable such as the orphan, the widow, the widower, the aged and those who lost their jobs from picking employments without welfare packages as casual workers since all of them could be forced to illicit works that would expose them to fatal injuries.

b) **BAN UNWHOLESOME GOODS:** All the substandard goods should be outlawed from the production and the distribution to the docile and illiterate consumers. No room for the expired products and in raw materials too in order to have quality goods in the marketplaces. These contaminated or expired goods include the consumables, materials for the building or constructions and those daily needs being used for the purpose of costume. The security workers at the ports should be at alert from clearing the inferior items to enter the nation. When the marketplaces are rid of the inferior goods that can maim the limbs and deaden the senses, then the incidence of increasing number of disability shall be minimal if not zero. In the words of the noblest *'avoid consuming all intoxicants even in its minutest'*. This is a word for a wise to prevent sending him into committing crimes against self and humanity.

c) **BUILD QUALITY INFRASTRUCTURES:** Zero tolerance to bad construction is a path to have accidents-free journey. All the building professionals should work in synergy from the plan stage to the commission stage. Certified professionals should manage and implement the building of the infrastructures.

d) **SAFETY KITS:** The laws of building of the factory premises should make it compulsory that no factory is open for use until all the safety kits are in the right places. The regulatory agencies must certify the kits are installed at the right places within and outside the factories before the certificate of the operation is awarded. Harsh punishment should be used to enforce that all institutions should be enforced to ensure the right things are done.

e) **END INFERIOR SERVICE:** All the services must be regulated to ensure that there is quality service from all the service providers. No projects that are of inferior standard should be commissioned. All the dilapidated structures should be demolished for the new ones with international best practices. Slums should be reconstructed to wear modern look for cheap logistics and location of houses and offices. It should be legislated that the quality tools are used for the constructions, the productions of goods and the services being rendered. Punitive measures against poor services shall eliminate indolence and unsatisfactory services.

f) **REJIG THE REGULATORY AGENCIES:** For the regulatory bodies in the nation to be effective and efficient, all the procurement of the human and non-human resources should be perfectly fit. All of them should work in synergy with the agencies that cater for the wellbeing of the citizens in order to ensure that they consume right.

g) **ZERO-GRAFT:** Impunity is the reason for the growth of corruption. The identified lacuna in justice dispensation should be worked upon to have zero-tolerance to graft in all shade, sizes and shapes across the boards.

h) **PROVISION FOR EMERGENCY:** There should be room for emergency when the need calls for it. This is the use of application approach. For instance, if the medical services are not appropriate or beyond the capacity of those in attendance, there should be numbers of professionals and the next door consultants that must be called to render assistance. Every street should have mobile clinic waiting for emergency calls. The mobile clinics and ambulance should be at strategic locations for the probable accidents victims. The roads should be accessorized with side roads clinics for emergency. There should be highly equipped emergency sections at the hospitals, primary, secondary and tertiary across the nooks and corners of the nation.

i) **HUMANITARIAN SERVICE:** People of all professions should be ever ready to render free social services to avoid the maiming of limbs and the loss of any part of the senses. There is nothing bad for volunteers who are conducting the movement of vehicles on the roads to prevent traffics of the motorists. Medical practitioners should be ready to assist someone in health crises along the road without being formally consulted. This humanitarian service revolves round the theme *'be your brother's keeper'*. Let every professional have it mind that they would render free service every day at any place and at any time. This free social and humanitarian service is their widow's mite.

j) **VOLUNTARY DONATIONS:** All should have the spirits of being philanthropists voluntary donating to impact lives and institutions. No amount of money donated to a charity is not valued and rewarded by God the Owner of all treasures and the Giver of riches. In fact, the best thing to do is always donate widow's mite if you do not have big pocket. The little shall fetch big returns here and there. I have seen a poor artisan that presented a fancy biro always used by a big customer of his for his birthday gifted. The rich man was so happy after the presentation that he awarded several tens of thousand contract job immediately to him. The biro was not up to five hundred naira.

k) **FINANCIAL EMPOWER:** Citizens who are not physically challenged could move up and down in search of funds and materials to support their business ideas unlike those who have some challenges that can hinder the movement. Therefore, government should earmark intervention funds for the use of the investors among the persons with special attention. The banks should devise a better way to fund the business ideas and the projects of the persons living with disabilities. The financing should have no collateral and practicable conditions. All other supports should be rendered including patronage of the goods and services of the persons. The people with the disabilities who have viable ideas should therefore reach out to those financial houses, the government agencies, the organizations and the likes who are offering the supports to start and build a business empire.The word 'ask' is a request and is not sinful. Let them politely ask, through the right channel of communication, for those who have the resources to provide the financial supports.

l) **SPECIAL CARE FOR THE AGED:** By this, we mean the vulnerable ones. The aged should enjoy right care. The quality health care is for all the citizens. Trained nurse, security attendants, basic needs care givers for the aged preparing the diet, the clothing and the bedding for the old, the counselor or psychologist, the comedian that can crack nice jokes to help the aged free from depression, psychotherapist and the book readers should be employed gratis for the aged. They should be under old age security or social security fund on monthly basis to relief the children. The numerical strength and other personal profile of the aged should be compiled by locations in order to provide the right aesthetics to live healthy and strong at the age.

m) **STUDY AND ACT INFORMATION:** Useful information are communicated through the medium of communication in this era of information and communication technology advancement should be used by the persons living with disabilities. Never ignore information as information is what all successful scholars, diplomats, technocrats and the likes have used to be what they are. Share the piece of information with others to improve your knowledge of ideas. Use all the relevant guides in prints and broadcast media for the development and the growth of your ambition. The use of certain prescriptions and the proscriptions could be a right guide to the top and the podium of honour. Use the senses and the working limbs right to be human assets that would positively add values to the national outputs.

n) **BE SELECTIVE:** It is not all the contents of any book is right for use. It is not all the information is worth useful for the involvement to add values to the gross domestic products hence the gross national income.

CHAPTER THREE

<u>EMPOWERING DISABLED: STAKEHOLDERS</u>

Preventing people from becoming handicapped is a topmost primary purpose of the government and the other stakeholders. Primarily, this must start from constitutional amendment in a way that the 'disable' is properly planned for ahead of time. If the constitution is re-written to accommodate social, economic and political needs of the disable, then their rights have been protected. For the disabled, none of their constitution-supported human rights must be trampled or infringed upon by any other citizen or foreigners, institution, establishments, pressure groups, association, under any guise. Therefore, the empowerment is started by the government. This is at outset done via implementing this approach of empowerment as the key to other provisions. This is the use of the Japanese popular proverb. What is the popular Japanese saying? It says *'give a man a fish and you have fed the man for a day, but instead teach him how to catch a fish and you have the man forever'*. This approach is inevitable to inculcate the right values, orientation, culture and right habits of self-development to the minds of the special people would rid the streets of beggars and sanitize the society at large. In addition to this as the basis of foundation to develop and nurture the talents and skills in the people, the government should lead the other stakeholders to get these done:

a) **UNVEIL VISTAS OF EMPLOYMENT OPPORTUNITIES:** Through the opening of new sectors from the existing sectors, new jobs from the existing jobs shall be created to engage the people living with disabilities to develop interest in. by the choices from the varieties of employment opportunities, supported with moral, legislative, technical and financial supports from the government and the stakeholders, the streets have been rid of beggars especially by the PLWDs. Instead of being beggars, they become philanthropists too from the legitimate income.

b) **PROMOTE THE NEW SECTORS:** People are reluctant to start a new business until they are convinced that the jobs are viable and could fetch them right size of income in profits. The consultants should be engaged to talk sense to the public focusing on the PLWDs in order to build their human capacity and develop interests for choice profession from the lists. The government should market the new jobs to them. For instance, in the modern world of developed digital technology, people can develop digital products and sell within their comfort zones. Cripple could develop varieties of digital books, digital advertisement, jingles, stickers, logos, cards and the likes for sale online. They could shop for used goods, procure at low prices and sell online again at higher prices from their homes. These should learn the need to run their business from their homes and other guides as contained in of our books 'Jobs with zero capital vol. 1 and 2.

c) **DE-EMPHASIZE CAPITAL TO START-UP:** The major challenge to the establishment of business by all entrepreneurs is the capital. Most businesses are capital intensive. The more the capital, the more the expansion of the business and the target profits. The solution is to teach the prospective entrepreneurs is to teach them how to start with little or zero capital. We introduced the use of the OPMs in the two-volume book *"Jobs with zero capital"*. The next step is the use of bootstrapping towards increasing the capital base. In a nation with poor financial management by the banks especially the failure of the apex bank and paucity of capital as a result of low earning in internally generated income, all should be taught on how to use bootstrapping.

d) **PROVISION OF MODERN INFRASTRUCTURES:** All the roads, rails and ports should take safety as primary. Both the workers and the users of the systems of transportation must be able to use safety machines for their movement of themselves and their assets. The right and relevant accessories must be at the right places and distances (points) to guide the users in order to prevent avoidable accidents. If it is possible, specially-built roads should be built for them. Special roads, rails and sea transportation should be built for the physically challenged.

e) **MODERN HEALTH FACILITIES:** The National Health Insurance Scheme (NHIS) should be pursued to ensure that all the citizens are captured in the scheme at low or subsidized cost. All the hospitals, private and the public owned, must be certified to have modern facilities and tools for the use of the patients. There should be zero excuse for failure to attend to the patients.

f) **MAXIMUM SECURITY ARCHITECTURE:** The security of lives and property is a primary function of governments at all levels. The parents and the communities must also take security as a major role to have a disabled-free society. Road marshals should synergize with the other security agencies to provide security for the citizens. Drunken driving, over speeding, the running of rickety vehicles that are malfunctioning engine and expired tyres on the wheel should be 'legislated' to be off the roads. Certified vehicles, trains, ships and airplanes that have met the right standards of quality should be allowed for transportation. The electronic devices for communication should not be substandard to avoid toxic emission that can lead to disability. Those managing the security architecture should be highly proficient and tolerating to all the races and religions in order to enjoy cooperation.

g) **INSURANCE:** There should be comprehensive insurance for every citizen since every able citizen is a potential handicapped by events and tides of life. Right legislation must be assented to for all companies and employers of labour to insure their workers in case of accidents that could lead to disabilities. All must be insured regardless of the age, gender, affiliation, places of residence in the nation and the likes.

h) **REGULATORY FUNCTIONS:** The regulatory bodies should ensure that all factories meet the standard in the availability of safety kits for the workers. The safety of the consumers should also be top priority. It is not just factories but all the importers should never import unwholesome goods to the nation which should a national duty and a combined task of the security agents and the regulatory agents at the ports. With these in mind, both the workers and the consumers are guaranty of quality health.

i) **EDUCATION:** One, education must be free and quality for the abled and the disabled. To produce the best in pupils, the native languages should be adopted to teach art, Mathematics, science and technology including history, civics education and the likes. Foreign language should be relegated to the communication purpose with other people from the other climes only. Two, there is the need to communicate what could harm people to avoid the accidents that could result in disability. Sensitization, through the use of mass media and other channels, must be high in the area of security and safety tips. All of them should enjoy free and quality special education from the government and the philanthropic organizations, education support bank should cater for the grants for the people living with disabilities. The special schools for them shall be a right ground to discover their talents and skills. At the schools, the potentials within are harnessed for the public patronage.

j) **SPECIAL ENDOWMENTS:** Public gathering and social interactions with the special people should be added in value with endowments purposely set up for the people. Stakeholders should inaugurate endowment funds for the specially challenged persons. Such endowments should be managed by quality persons, trustworthy with epitome of exemplary character. They must be celebrated like the others.

k) **TRUST FUND:** There should be legislated supports for the intervention fund for the PLWDs. Special trust funds should therefore be put in place for the disable to access from the designated banks. The donors to the accounts should be from all the stakeholders led by the government. The funds can gain added values by individuals and institutions.

l) **SPORTS AND TRAINING ACTIVITIES:** The sports complex should be accommodating to the people living with challenges in order to be able to have the facilities used for practicing or training like the able-body people.

m) **SPECIAL TRANSPORTATION:** This is the challenge before the auto-investors and designers to design such cars and vehicles that would be easy for the transportation of the PLWDs. By this, the facilities in the public transportation sector should be fabricated in a way that the cripple would find it easy to enter the public transport. The blind should be able to find their ways to the bus stop. The deaf and dumb should be able to communicate and enjoy the social services.

n) **PUBLIC POST APPOINTMENTS:** There should be no room for discrimination on the right to apply for any public and private jobs. It is onus on the government to create right environment in offices that are equipped with right tools that would help them to be active and efficient in the public service. The blind should be supported with braille materials to work on certain files. The cripple should be able to wheel themselves to the offices at ground floors. The right of the able-body workers should also be for the disabled working in the public and private sectors. Only the works that require frequent movement from place to place, office to office should be left only for the able-body workers. Certain clerical jobs should be left for the special people with all the accessories that would help them deliver on the job. A certain percentage for the PLWDs should be legislated in the national constitution.

o) **PATRONAGE:** Government should be the major patrons of the products and services of the citizens particularly the people living with disabilities. By studies, the failure of government to add values to the productions from the entrepreneurs has become the reason for the low profits and decline in productivity. If government creates silos and engages in farms to stores where government earmarks budgets on annual basis to procure all the farm produce from the farmers and then resells at lower prices to the consumers, there would be higher outputs from the farmers for the silos.

p) **DEFINED CONTRIBUTION PLAN:** All the PLWDs should be keyed into such pension scheme whether they are employed by the private or the public enterprise. The step is to prepare them for the future in order to be free from financial crises. It is a plan for the rainy days since administrative and legislative policies in the future may not favour the aged care funding from the coffers of the nation especially if the nation has lower revenue generation base.

q) **OLD AGE BENEFITS:** Aside the palliative measures for them in the wake of financial losses in business, there should be 'severance packages' for them as retiree benefits from the government even though they were never public servants. Such benefits could be a stipend as social fund on monthly basis and free treatments at the public and private hospitals.

r) **FISCAL ALLOCATION:** The persons living with disabilities should have budgetary allocation on annual basis to cater as financial provision for their social and economic needs.

s) **AWARDS RECOGNITION:** Government should lead the packs that must recognize their mettle in different areas of life endeavours. All the associations, institutions and individuals who are wealthy should recognize their inputs to the nation and the registering of the nation in the world map.

MOTIVATING DISABLED

Motivation starts from self. They must lift self from the level of begging. All the disabled persons should have **self-motivation** in order to face the challenges squarely without transferring their personal issues on others as human liabilities. We have seen people that are engaging in artisanal jobs such as tailoring, shoe repairing, barbing, braiding, bead making, costumier and the likes. The elites among them are in classrooms teaching on wheelchairs like the popular and bestselling author, erudite scholar, diplomat and award-winning writer, Professor **Chinualumogu Achebes** of this world. Several jobs are office jobs that can be practised by the people with physical challenges. We have seen specialized lawyers, doctors, engineers, architects, surveyors, marketers, administrators and the likes who employ people to work for them. Towards self-motivation, the PLWDs must also do the following:

a) **READ:** There is no time wasting in reading books. Reading is knowledge searching and a path to grow intellectually and learn to kill or suppress depression. There is no way that a person would not fall into depression in one thing or the other. Everyone, no matter one's state of health, amount of wealth, quality of social resources, the position of authority, the status, the social esteem, the degree of popularity, the level of piety among countless reasons and features, should prepare to find time to read with the mindset to find practicable solutions to depression. Authors write on different issues to increase the spirituality of the readers. In books are invaluable lessons and eyes openers to vistas of opportunities contained in free information released through the print, broadcast and electronic media by the technocrats. In my book '*Wastes to wealth jobs*', we revealed how people can identify jobs from reading the newspaper, watching television and surfing the internet. Through reading tomes of selected books shall advance the knowledge and exposure of the readers who are called book worms. Inside the print at a leisure place of comfort, one traverses the earth and the whole universe unless one decides to limit one's scope of learning and exposure to facts and figures about life and the environments. Reading varieties of books from different authors and publishing companies including the daily or weekend newspapers should become a hobby. Read biographies. Read the intellectual presentations in columns and feature writing inside prints for critical studies. Employ someone who could read to learn from the texts. Read editorials from the editors of newspapers. Think deeply from the forewords and preface from book reviewers. After reading, writing becomes the next line of action to increase the wisdom, intelligence and knowledge from the exposure through the perusal of books. Tomes of books should be read by the persons at their comfort zones in order to boost the knowledge. Varieties of books should be read in other to have vast knowledge on all issues. If it is possible, read a book at least a week. Share what you read to have greater understanding for easy application of the contents.

b) **LISTEN TO RADIO:** On radio programmes are varieties of educative, informative and instructional contents that can bring the best out of listeners. Interactions on radio and the brainstorming of contributors on the radio as feedbacks and respondents help to develop the intellectual capacity of the listeners. Listen to conversations and interviews from professionals and scholars on the mass media to add values to the knowledge and wisdom. This shall advance the speech making and writing.

c) **WATCH THE TELEVISION:**Watching the terrestrial and cable television enables the watcher to travel wider for the audio visual productions. Therefore, for the immense gains, create time to watch the documentaries and the broadcast stuffs from the television station, terrestrial and cable. Keen watchers of programmes on the tube shall learn a big deal. In fact, the contents from different producers are motivators and eyes openers to new things and open vistas of opportunities.

d) **SURF INTERNET:** Browse internets through the regular visits and travel round the world from your comfort zones. The internet is like a 'seer' or 'spiritual messenger' expecting you to ask for anything in information. The developers have developed apps that would proffer solutions to your questions at the press of buttons within a few seconds. Internet via search engine optimizations is a craze in town for every enthusiast who desires to be abreast of world events from the corners of one's home and office. Improve the knowledge and skills with the access to computer packages and the information. With right information, opportunities are unveiled and identified for personal development.

e) **USE THE INFORMATION:** From the reads and the information sourced on internet, the next stage is to use them for self-development. The style of bestseller writers and award winning films and songs including poetries learnt from the books and the internet shall add values to the outputs from the persons.

f) **TEACH OTHERS:** Never by miserly in your behavior. Be prepared to share what you have in order to have more as recompense. Sharing knowledge is a way to have fuller understanding of issues especially in the formulation of practicable solutions to social and other problems. Teaching is impacting others and spreading the knowledge to add greater values to the nation at large.

g) **SELF-TUTORING:** One should stop at where the teachers stop, there should be crave for seeking more knowledge. A good pupil consults series of supplementary books to add greater value to the acquired knowledge. One should never see self as 'Mr. know all' but rather 'Mr. seek all' to be able to have vast knowledge about things. Every humble, brilliant and intelligent teacher has a teacher or even teachers. By this, every teacher is a pupil vice versa. Never stop learning after taking notes from your tutor or mentor. Revise and review what you have learnt. Learn to ask about what you do not know. Ask and people shall guide you to the right knowledge. Asking is part of learning and improving the intelligence and wisdom. The noblest says *'learning is from cradle to grave'*.

h) **HAVE A MENTOR:** Be patience and considerate to pick your mentor. The mentor could be seasoned teacher or a consultant. Consult those who know to boost your areas of interest. Mentors are proud to facilitate progress from the mentees. The right products from a mentor are pride to the mentor. Who would not be proud of his quality mentee?

i) **STRIVE TO BE ROLE MODEL:** In your attitude while learning new things to add values to what you have, strive to live a model life as mirror to others. In the community you resident, you are a model to many. Protect your name by minding your character and temperament. Live with the three T's namely trustworthy, truthful and transparent in all the dealings with different people at all places on all issues.

j) **BE PIOUS:** This is where the religion tenets and precepts come into play. None is from no source. No man drops from heavens. Every creature has a creator and that is God. For man living with disability to have tranquility, piety of the prescriptions and the proscriptions of the almighty shall serve the purpose of becoming pious. God does not look at the face and physical ability but what runs in the mind that is done with the limbs. Live a pure heart in order to live a righteous life.

k) **FORM OR JOIN A CLUB:** They should have places and time of social activities for the, to relax their brains and limbs in social club. They could have theirs and endeavor to join any social club where they can also contribute to the society and the nation. There is barrier stopping them from joining all the professional and societal association where they can contribute their own quotas to the society and the nation at large. In schools, the alma mater should be one of the associations they should be active members.

l) **JOIN RIGHT FORUM OR GROUP:** Group chats help to discover hidden talents and vistas of opportunities. Join the online discussions on all the media houses, print, broadcasting, electronic or social media. We are in an era where digital technology plays major role in the development of self and promoting products and services from one's comfort stations.

The second **motivation** to the people living with disabilities could be said to come from the government. Government should create level playing field for them to achieve their future goals for their vision and mission to be accomplished. The popular maxim says 'a sauce for goose is a sauce for gander'. Every citizen, regardless of the age, status, affiliations and physical capability should enjoin equal treatment in the resources sharing and allocations. Periodic national constitutional review in support of the disabled and the communication of the rights which they have access to enjoy is a motivating movement. We have several measures to motivate the physically and mentally challenged into being creative. Some of these are:

a) **LEARNING TOOLS:** Those living with impaired eyes, slur brains and the bad hearing should be supported by the relevant devices that would enhance the senses to be working. They should have free access to the tools to aid their movement, aid their speech making, allow perfect understanding and enliven their memories as the advancement in technologies improve. Professor **Chinualumogu Albert Achebe** taught between 1991 and 2009 at Bard College after the provision of the relevant tools that would assist him on teaching job. This is a good lesson for all the employers of people with disabilities. It is like creating right workplace environment for effectiveness and efficiency of the special persons. In short, the learning tools include the well-stocked libraries, conventional and e-book libraries for the use of the users.

b) **SPECIAL SCHOOLS:** The special schools should be reachable to the target beneficiaries. As a school age pupil, what we saw at school at the first day endeared the love of being a pupil in the school. The structure and the facilities should be attractive for the target pupils. The special schools should be adequately equipped with teaching and learning aids and kits including the instructional materials for the stakeholders for easier disseminating of knowledge for scholars, diplomats, technocrats and the likes to be produced amongst the PLWDs. There should be equipped libraries with relevant books that would impact them positively and create entrepreneurial spirits in them. Relevant laboratories should be in the schools. The curriculums and the extra curriculum activities should be highly sensitive to the development and growth of their health and mental capacity. Instead of having mushroom schools that are not tailored towards teaching and researching for the people requiring special attentions, all the people living with disabilities should have their schools with all disabilities in a learning environment for proper integration and mutual understanding of one another.

c) **MENTORING:** One of the ways to empower and motivate the people is through the right mentoring. All the sections of the people living with disabilities would regain their self-esteem and build confidence to be active in what they have in business ideas. If the music stars who are disabled are sponsored to talk to them, many would see no hindrance in being popular musicians with chart topper songs. Professionals like the disabled lawyers, disabled doctors, veteran or seasoned broadcaster, chartered accountants, brilliant academics, successful businessmen with one disability or the other shall be right mentors for them to think outside the box in order to be economically and financially independent.

d) **SPECIAL CONSULTANTS:** Counseling of the people shall add right values to the special people with the special needs. All the schools of the handicapped and the vulnerable people at welfare homes should have visiting consultants on transformation and rehabilitation of the people in order to integrate them with the public.

e) **SPECIAL FUNDING:** People with special needs must be able to access funds for the creativities they have in mind to pursue. The financial institutions, the philanthropic organizations, the right agencies of government could and should make funds available for the people for investment with zero conditions of repayment. Intervention funds and grants for the PLWDs shall motivate them into doing something meaningful to impact the nation and the fellow citizens without becoming human burdens on them. Just as the nation has certain percentage is earmarked for the education like the former Education Tax Fund now the Tertiary Education Trust Fund (TETFUND) from the business organization and the government, there is a need to have special trust funds for the people living with disabilities to fund their inventions and ideas in order to add values to the national economy.

f) **PATRONAGE:** It is operation buy what they produce and pay handsomely for their services. If the federal government could use recent Presidential Executive Orders 003 (PEO3) to enjoin the Ministries, Departments and Agencies to patronize all the locally made goods, then this should be communicated and interpreted to include the products and services of the people living with disabilities. All makers of products require patronage of products and services especially from the government and the community in general in order to make profits. In fact, this efforts if done religiously shall improve both micro and macro economy of the nation and improve the values of the legal tender. By so doing, the deficit in the balance of trade shall be of little effect from its decline.

g) **EMPLOYMENT OPORTUNITIES:** These should be employed into the civil service jobs with all the facilities that would enhance their effectiveness and efficiency on the jobs. Although the percentage of the people living with disabilities are small, the percentage should be scaled up and communicated to them at the special schools as a way to motivate them into passing with flying colours in their choice courses of studies.

h) **NO STIGMATIZATION:** All the PLWDs are people of integrity, dignity and reverence that should be treated with decency and respect. Physical disability does not mean mental disability, sexual performance disability and others. The public must never deprive them of any right. Marry them and marry them out to others. Respect their views in the community. Let them have their say and way politely examined for adoption. Never open room for their deprivation and failures to make impact. Always create room for their excellent performance with right incentives and motivations. No one should use libelous and offensive languages against them in private and public places. Every human being is honourable and deserves right humane treatment who deserve right assistance at the time of needs. There should be zero room for stigmatization of those living with disabilities in offices, rooms and public places. Equal opportunities should be given to the people to avoid treating them like the second citizens in the societies they are found. Relevant bills should be passed by the national and state assemblies on the halt of discrimination against the people with disabilities by the parents, the siblings, the relatives, friends and the residents in the community. The mottos should either be *'what an able person can do, the disable can also do'* or *'fundamental human right is human right for all regardless of the ability and disabilities'*. Government, associations, institutions and individuals can institute fundamental right actions against those who intentionally infringe on the rights of the people living with disabilities.

i) **RECOGNITIONS:** Awards for recognitions should be instituted for the achievers among the people living with one disability or the other periodically. All the personalities should be therefore periodically recognized for their contribution to the society especially in the inputs to the national outputs across all the sectors.

j) **SPORTS COMPETITIONS:** They should be engaged in sports contests that would serve as the meeting points. Such special sports should be organized in the same manner the sports for the able body people is organized. In the recent, there was amputee world football competition at Mexico. Olympic Games have Paralympics games for the people living with disabilities. This is a motivation for the persons to have a sense of belonging and integrate themselves to the system. It serves as a way to end stigmatization of the people with special needs.

k) **SOCIAL FUND:** By legislative and executive orders, all the people with one form of disability or the other should be on the payroll of the government and philanthropic organization. Certain percentage of the corporate social responsibility funds should be set apart to fund the projects and human capacity building of the people with special needs. Direct funding of the structures of the schools of the special people should be legislated in the national assembly and domiciled by the states in the federation.

l) **NEITHER ABUSE NOR TRAMPLE ON THEIR HUMAN RIGHTS:** A part of approach morally to empower the physical challenged is never to scorn at them. They should be treated with care and love. In fact, they should be the first to be attended to in any gathering. At public places, they should be assisted to enjoy the utilities before the others who are capable. All the staff of banks should be willing to assist them for the banking transactional services before the able-body customers.

m) **FREE LITIGATION:** They should enjoy pro bono representations at the court where they seek redress injustice and fight for the rights some had trampled upon at the courts of jurisdictions. The state attorney-general and minister of justice should prepare good prosecutors or defense counsel, depending on the matter, for them whenever they press charges against oppressors or others who had infringed on their rights at the courts of jurisdiction. Another area of strength to support the persons living with disabilities is the rolling out of **RIGHT LEGISLATION.** Periodically, the legislation should be reviewed to suit the people in the environment in a way to proffer solutions to the social, economic, technological and political issues. These acts should provide free and quality education to all the people living with disabilities.

n) **FREE SOCIAL SERVICES:** If the people without any form of disability could stand up against the government over freebies like the free education, free health care services and the likes, the people living with disabilities have more from the government and the other stakeholders.

o) **RE-ORIENTATION:** There is the need to re-orientate people living with disability to discard the bad culture that pushes them into low self-esteem and begging to sustain their needs through periodical motivational talks organized by the government, religion and business organizations and philanthropic bodies, individuals and groups. All of them should have self-belief to achieve greats in life. The spirit of 'I can' or 'I will' should be inculcated in them. The society should enhance their thinking and the level of contributions to the societies they are found. All should be able to speak their minds in the midst of other people. And their thoughts and sayings should be respected.

p) **NO VOTING DISENFRANCHISEMENT:** The eligible voters are for the citizens of eighteen years and above by the electoral laws. The PLWDs should be able to vote for candidates and parties of their choices at the time and places of voting. This is a respect for the voting right to avoid disenfranchisement. All deserve due respect and standpoints on issues. Respect is said to be reciprocal. They should have their saying and in many times their ways. They have rights to vote and be voted for to hold the public offices. It is onus on the government and the community stakeholders to put in place right tools and devices that would allow them to be active in politics. The recent introduction of the braille balloting for the people with visual challenges to vote is a right step towards the right direction. We have suggested the use of e-voting in some of our publications for the people including the PLWDs to vote at their comfort zones. The use of just three passwords and select the party of choice or candidates of choice on the mobile phones shall reduce the stress of the voters especially the physically challenged people. The three passwords have information that would disqualify the non-eligible voters who are those below eighteen years, non-citizens and multiple voting. The Bank Verification Number (BVN), the registered Mobile Phone Number (MPN) and the Permanent Voter Card(PVC) code number. If there is fraud in the data supplied especially in the birthday and nationality, such has disqualified self from participation.

q) **FEEL BELONGING:** None should be ostracized for their disability or disabilities. All are created as human beings with protected civil rights. The PLWDs should have their own associations too where they have their rights discussed. They should be active contributors to the national and global issues. In the associations, there should be communiqué releases for the government and the other stakeholders to acknowledge and work upon.

r) **TRAINING AND SCALING UP:** As a result of inability to have all the required information and tools for services, the government leading the other stakeholders should offer periodic free training and how to scale up their capacity with freebies. Just like every other entrepreneur or self-reliant citizen, periodical trainings on the job or choice profession shall be added values to the outputs from their workplaces.

s) **WORK AND WORKPLACE ETIQUETTES:** By this, we need to educate them on workplace etiquettes too in order to be abreast of required information to scale through possible hurdles in the course of doing their choice profession. Right materials should be presented to them for easy understanding of what to do at what time and places.

t) **MOTIVATION:** Every person requires motivations to achieve set dream or goals. Learning from the histories of the successful entrepreneurs is a right path. **Henry Ford** was reported to have gone broke five times before he founded Ford Motor. **Bill Gates** of Microsoft Incorporation fame fails with his first business, Traf-O-Data. **Steve Jobs** was kicked out of Apple yet he became one of the greatest inventors in the combined technology and art invented devices. The persons living with disabilities should have their mindset trained to be positive in order to make breakthrough in the chosen careers.

CHAPTER FOUR

<u>RIGHT ENVIRONMENT FOR DISABLED</u>

By this, we shall talk about factory aesthetics which the people should work at. It is constitutional for all to pay their taxes. The people living with disabilities could be helped to become entrepreneurs by the following provisions:

a) **PARENTING:** Parents are the role models and mentors to the children who teach the children about life and what it takes to live a quality life by their acts and sayings. All these teachings on how the children could identify problems and proffer solutions in order to be free from depression shall prepare the children for the challenges in any relationship in the school, streets, offices, matrimonial homes and the public in general There should be right environment at homes where the child is trained on how to be responsible and hardworking. The parents must not live a depressed life in order to produce right children with right frame of mindset. This is a must as depression is transferable and could lead to self-inflict disabilities. A home should also have right facilities such as library that must be well stocked with relevant books and illustrative charts. Parents must create future entrepreneurs from the four walls of homes under the watchful guidance of the parents. The primary roles of the parents are beyond the basic needs but including building futures from the home.

b) **ENABLING SOCIAL ENVIRONMENT:** Every citizen that is targeting to be entrepreneur requires right social environment. The people living with disabilities should not be exposed to insecure environment. By insecurity, since they have right and freedom to religion too, they must not be settled or allotted a location of business at insecurity-prone areas. This is a reason for the consultants to work with them from the development of their business proposals to the implementation.

c) **NATIONAL INVESTMENT PROMOTION COMMISSION ACT:** With the amendments to the Nigerian Investment Promotion Commission Acts which incorporate those with certain disability, then all the people living with disabilities would enjoy business protections and free from unhealthy promotion against their products and services. The export-import institutions (bank and administrative) should support the production of the creative PLWDs.

d) **UTILITIES AT THEIR BECK AND CALL:** There must be utilities at the press of a button for the people that are physically challenged. Through the access to the public utilities, they are free from depression and high costs of production. If it is possible, they should enjoy subsidies on the bills for all the utilities.

e) **RIGHT BUSINESS SCHOOLS:** For the nation to be free from the issue of unemployment, the school curriculum or syllabi should be reviewed in a way that all the subjects or courses of studies should be re-written in a way to produce vocational and technical graduates that can be self-reliance or self-employ themselves after graduation. All schools should not be ill-equipped, the teachers and non-teaching staffers should never be ill-motivated in order to get the right result in quality manpower who can be on their own. Through the special schools, teaching, researching and consultancy shall be easily achieved by the special people. Many of them could be vocational and technical sound to scale up the clients base across the boards.

f) **SPECIAL BANKS:** It is high time the nation opened such banks like Education Support Banks for the students regardless of their abilities and disabilities to seek for interest-free loans. The PWLDs must be treated like every other person with access to the loans for the studying of choice courses. The access to loans shall be a good avenue to build entrepreneurs among them from the schools.

g) **ACCESS TO THE L'S AND M'S:** They should have cheap access to the land, labour and loan at their comfort zones since what the able-body persons can do through movements to any place at designed times, they could not do the same. Government and the other stakeholders should render assistance for the processing of the inputs for productions.

h) **LOW TAXES:** All causes of depression and low esteem should be avoided by all the stakeholders. They must be subjected to develop high blood pressure as entrepreneurs. For beginners among the persons, zero tax or tax holiday could be adopted as taxation policy in order to cut the costs of production as a way of motivating them into productivity.

i) **FASTER BUREAUCRACY:** If it possible, they should be given online and home services for the bureaucracy to have no effect on what they are planning to do. The fast bureaucracy shall add values to the outputs of the persons with such disabilities.

j) **WORKING TOOLS:** All the modern work tools that would make the work faster and of quality should also be cheaply accessed through outsourcing. The cheap logistic environment shall add values to the outputs of these people.

k) **RIGHT MARKETPLACES:** The investment on the e-commerce by improved investment on information and communication technology shall add value to the outputs from all entrepreneurs particularly the people living with disabilities. For the publishers and authors, reading culture must be improved upon for the promotion and distribution of the intellectual property. The works should tour schools and the book markets like book fairs to have right size of sales.

INPUT: OUTPUT BY THE DISABLED

By this, we pray the people living with disabilities should break out of their shells and become employments creators instead of turning themselves into human liabilities. The challenges being faced by people and the other things in the environment are enough to create jobs and nurse viable business ideas. The perfect uses of the senses determine the level of output from the disabled. The **policy formulation** on industrialization from the policy makers of the government shall add right values to the outputs from the disabled. The new policy should identify with the people living with disabilities in the establishment of their business ideas. All the sectors of the economy must be strengthened to accommodate them. With all the cited ways to empower and motivate them to high level of performance earlier, there is increased input (involvement) and output of international best practice.

Nevertheless, the disabled should not anticipate a perfect business operating environment before thinking on viable ideas they can work upon in order to be self-reliant. The stress of getting jobs or competing with others who are without defects should be a motivation to start their own businesses with the available facilities and inputs at their beck and call. By the pervading state of things, human wants and needs are unlimited. The gaps must be continually filled by the combined efforts of the people with disability in order to grow the economy.All the persons living with disabilities have opportunities to become artpreneurs like artists, e-artist, sculptor, carvers, weavers, braiders, repairers, technopreneurs with quality skills in information and communication technology, business entrepreneurs, e-marketers or e-advertisers, tutors and several others in administrative, social service jobs, technical-based, cultural-based and commercial based jobs from the basis of choices and areas of interests by the innate skills and talents. There are other jobs the people who have physical challenges can engage in to increase the national output with little or no support. Some of these products and services from the comforts of the homes of the disabled are:

a) **WRITINGBUSINESS:** This comprises authoring of books, journals, news reporting, film scripting, proof reading and the likes. A writer must be up to date in information to communicate maximally with his or her target audience. There is no writer that can exhaust what to write about. Issues crop up every day for people who have interest to write to script in books and printable materials. The publishing is a vast business that has paved the way for productions in films, documentaries and audio-products in audio books. In fact, no one can exhaust what to write about till eternity.

b) **DRAWING:** This is an imaginative business that shows creativity of the doers. Cartoon, illustrative artworks and the likes are some of the business activities such should be able to do without stress.

c) **ACTING:** In the popular films, many people living with disabilities are prominently featured and they acted wonderfully. The script writers of such blockbuster films could be people living with disabilities too who featured the disabled in order to give right recognition to the people in the society.

d) **DESIGNINGTRADE:** Creative fashion designers are from PLWDs since the brains is the sensitive part of the body transcribed by the hands. We can include packaging and branding to this for the creative and intelligent persons living with disabilities. This also includes giftware business that can be done at the comfort zones of the PLWDs. The level of creativity would determine the aesthetics and branding.

e) **AUDITING BUSINESS:** This is clerical office job where the keen analysis of the records is the prerequisite to be efficient. There are persons living with disabilities that have the educational qualifications to run home-office auditing job as a private operators.

f) **MARKETING AND ADVERTISING:** From one's comfort zones especially of the PLWDs, they could invent jingles for commercials on the media to promote a product or service to others.

g) **E-BUSINESS:** In the world today, one of the gains of the advanced digital and internet technology is the buying and selling online. This is a business that is open to everybody. At least, if one does not have a product or service to sell, one must have knowledge of those makers and service providers that require independent sellers or sales agents. Impacted internet and digital skill knowledge on them shall transform them into busy bees earning legitimately from the internet innovations and the use of the devices.

h) **ORATORICAL BUSINESS:** Speech making is a viable business that can transform many into substance in life. Many have good voices that are good for communicators. Today, many are seasoned on air personalities in the popular communication media stations. There are seasoned and intelligent poets among the people with disabilities.

i) **MOTIVATION SPEAKING:** We have used the example of **John Foppe**at the early part of the book who is a motivational speaker and earning big from the public speaking business. Such presentation can turn them into speech writers, editors and the likes.

j) **MASTER OF CEREMONY:** There are ceremonies that featured people who are vocal and charismatic in speech making in the public as comperes. Many of the prophets who are blind are always sound and brilliant by the level of natural intelligence. Studies confirm that blind people have greater emotional intelligence. Those who are funny could become comedians cracking jokes at social engagements for a fee. Creating side attractions is a lucrative job in parties.

k) **VALUE ADDED CHAINS BUSINESSES:** All the producers of goods and service providers have products with long value chains in by-products that are convertible to other useful products. There are products from farms that be transformed into other consumables from the kitchens. As a writer, many of my books are triggered by the interviews and featured writings. Contents of books can be acted in films and documentaries. Motivational books can be acted and used to educate audience. Problems facing different strata have catalyzed the publication of books, production of films and research materials. There is no product an able person can do that cannot be done by the disabled.

GDP AND GNI IN RELATIONSHIP WITH THE DISABLED

At outset under 'introduction', we highlighted some people that suffered certain disability that are wealthy. Many of them are multimillionaires in assets and net worth. There are billionaires among them. From the bottom, they reach the top. It was a journey of nothing to something that influenced others. The histories do not show that they begged to live quality lives. They never relied on the parents or guardians to be substance in life. They rise from grass to grace without allowing their disabilities to low their spirits to be successful in their endeavours. This is a good path and suffices as a model for those begging for survival. In self-motivation with the supports from all the stakeholders, the growth in the gross domestic products and the gross national income is inevitable from the large number living with disabilities.

Being disabled is inability. Everyone has potentials to nurture. Disability is never inability. We are all stakeholders as we are all prone to disabilities by our actions and inactions. The failure of an institution or the fellow human beings could have negative effect on our lives. Depression comes in different forms and sizes which must be fought headlong by proffering the right solutions in anticipation. As the abled persons by physical and mental state can fall into depression, likewise the persons living with disabilities can. All hands must therefore be on deck to fight back depression. And depression that could lead to further woes or increase the state of mental and physical disability is solved by finding the exact opposite of our challenges. If a job loss is the cause of your depression, seek for another job. If sexual deprivation by your cheating spouse led to your depression, find a mentor and marriage counselor or talk it over with your spouse or find alternative to replace your sexual urge. If failure to win a job, lead a team to a successful end, win a hand in marriage, to have a well-bred and brilliant children after heavy spending on their education and the basic needs, failure to win in an election after all the resources expended, failure win a case despite the exhibits presented at the courts of jurisdiction, financial loss of sales on your best products or services, failure to earn right royalties for your intellectual property, failure to meet the set standard despite all your inputs, failure to have your rights protected but instead being trampled upon by the oppressors…. All these could lead to depression which may lead to greater disability. Disabuse your mind with the maxim *'que serai serai'* literally meaning *'what will be will be'* of the Latin. Let the verses from the incorruptible scriptures be in your mind and brain at every time and places where frustrations have set in. what are these golden verses? '<u>Do not say we believe, we believe and that you would not be tested. WE tested those before you. You shall surely undergo test in order to sieve the true believers from the fake believers</u>" and the second reveals "<u>Verily, WE shall test you with fear (insecurity), hunger (deprivation of food, sex, basic and social needs), loss of lives (to sudden death) loss of goods (decline in resources) loss of fruits (personal gains from disasters)</u>.But, where is the solution? The solution is at the tail end of the verses '<u>those who admit that everything is from God and to HIM is the return,</u>

In retrospect, one must not just resign himself to fate but strive towards living a decent life by observing the do's and don'ts in order to have self-fulfillment. Anticipate depression that could sneak in your life in any form. Brace up to have readily made solutions. This is an anticipated approach and you should never apply '*wait and see approach*' to suppress all forms and sizes of depression which creates the largest percentage of disabilities. Every stakeholder should be up to the task to prevent accidents and incidents that could lead to disabilities. Government must be responsive and live to their primary and secondary responsibilities. Everyone must play the roles assigned or bestowed on him and her. We should all be optimistic about life and hence the need to plan ahead. Through empathy, we should continually donate to the wellbeing of the persons living with disabilities since majority of them are never born with any disability. We are therefore potential disable till we breathe our last. Every man is capable of building mansion on the skies regardless of the state of the physical fitness. Never give up hope. Be courageous to move on in life. Life is never static. It is a transient. There is no permanent stage in life. Discover your natural endowment and horn the inborn talent. Develop interest in skill and artisanal jobs. Adopt a mentor for the area of interest. Read the right materials that would enhance your interested profession. Rub minds with people with high intelligent quotient or intellectual capacity. Build friendship with people of great thought and vision. Add values to your personality through right associations. Contribute your intellectual reasoning on public issues. Popularize your person by joining the right group on social media. Respond to issue with wisdom and intelligence. People shall respect you with the caliber of personalities you associate with. Build interest in a skill and start something. Loss of senses is never an obstacle to grow innate ideas as done in the saner climes. Avoid all the causes of depression to lower the number of people that would suffer from disabilities hence state the budget for the persons living with disabilities.

"Work on depression, a major cause of disability
Life is never a bed of roses
Anticipate challenges and practicable solutions
No challenge exists without solutions
Beside each problem are its solutions
Choose your choice solution and move on
Live a life of moderation
High hope is being ambitious
Regardless of the capability and ability
Especially the degree of sense and limbs

Being blind does not open room for begging
Your dignity and integrity is always at stake
Enroll to learn the use of braille
Use braille devices to broad knowledge
Develop interest in choice skills
Read to become writer and thespian
And you earn right royalty for your work
Being armless does not send you to the street begging to survive
Armless **John Foppe** is earning big as speech speaker at functions
Armless could use his charismatic voice to be motivational speaking
Being cripple is suffice to learn a skill in building and repairing
Being a deaf and dumb never pushed any to begging
Learn a trade with your eyes and brains in proper use
Opportunities are there in e-commerce
Open your brains to by-products to work on
Add value to the secondary values of the primary products
It is a trade in the products and services of others

Never bury your talents in the soil
Horn your talents to empower self, community and nation"

<u>**ABOUT THE BOOK**</u>

There are books for the people living with physical challenges in different economies showing how to add values to them hence they contribute to the national economy from deficit spending and high rate of unemployment to surplus budget. Biting economies of nations have pushed many of the persons with disabilities into begging for sustenance. By studies, majority of the people living with disabilities are products of self-inflict, midwives' negligence and complications during child births. By studies, only a few are genuinely born with disabilities. Epidemics of diseases have resulted into disabilities and malfunctioned of the parts of the body. The failure in the primary responsibilities of the government and the other stakeholders has led to the loss of limbs and memories of the citizens. Yet, by critical studies, all human beings have natural endowments that can scale up the national output if right measures are put in place for the supports of the persons living with disabilities. For all the inborn resources to be able to complement the environmental resources, all hands must therefore be on deck by all the stakeholders led by the government by the contents of the book written in a very lucid English language. The book further espouses how people can live normally without living with disabilities, what should be installed for their efficiency by their employers, how those living with deformity can regain their self-confidence and build their choice careers as entrepreneurs or self-reliant personalities like the others without any disability. We therefore deemed it fit to put together how these could add values to the national output by the increase of the gross domestic products in order to shore up what can be budgeted for the social service sectors to improve the standard of living. At this juncture, the contents place emphases on what can be done to bring the best out of the physically challenged ones in the societies cum nation.

<u>**ABOUT THE AUTHOR**</u>

Author **Amusa Abdulateef** is a talented and inspirational writer who has authored **over sixty international books** on different issues targeting at proffering solutions to all national and international issues as Mr. 'Trouble Shooter'. Based on researches and studies, he, as a prolific writer, child educationist, motivational speaker, socio-economic researcher, writer of all literary genres for different categories of readers, public analyst and an administrator has impact lives and institutions by his intellectual resources in books and seminars papers. He is a product of the citadel of technological innovation, The Polytechnic, Ibadan Nigeria where he graduated as a business administrator; married and blessed with lively children.

OTHER BOOKS FROM THE AUTHOR

Amusa Abdulateef (2018) **Habits** CreateSpace Independent Publishing USA

Ditto (2018) **Intimate Domestic Violence** CreateSpace Publishing Industry USA

Ditto (2017) **In the hard times** CreateSpace Publishing Industry USA

Ditto (2017) **Words are absolutely powerful**CreateSpace Publishing Industry USA

Ditto (2017) **Securing the world through the youths**CreateSpace Publishing Industry USA

Ditto (2018) **Zero Depression**CreateSpace Publishing Industry USA

Ditto (2018) **Ask**CreateSpace Publishing Industry USA

Ditto (2018) **Hate Speech**CreateSpace Publishing Industry USA

Ditto (2017) **Words Are Absolutely Powerful** CreateSpace Publishing Industry USA

Ditto (2017) **Enabling Business Environment..** CreateSpace Independent Publishing USA

Ditto (2013) **Creating new jobs from the existing jobs** Iuniverse Publishing Company USA

Ditto (2012) **Jobs with zero capital vol. one** AuthorHouse Publishing Company USA

www.ingramcontent.com/pod-product-compliance
Lightning Source LLC
Chambersburg PA
CBHW031154250726
48655CB00002B/962